100 Hand Cases

100 Hand Cases

Martin I. Boyer, MD, FRCS(C)

Carol B. and Jerome T. Loeb Professor of Orthopedic Surgery,
Co-Chief, Hand and Wrist Service,
Washington University School of Medicine,
St. Louis, Missouri

James Chang, MD, FACS

The Johnson & Johnson Distinguished Professor of Surgery
and Orthopedic Surgery,
Chief, Division of Plastic and Reconstructive Surgery,
Stanford University School of Medicine,
Stanford, California

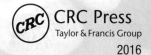

CRC Press
Taylor & Francis Group

2016

CRC Press
Taylor & Francis Group
6000 Broken Sound Parkway NW, Suite 300
Boca Raton, FL 33487-2742

© 2016 by Taylor & Francis Group, LLC
CRC Press is an imprint of Taylor & Francis Group, an Informa business

No claim to original U.S. Government works

Printed on acid-free paper
Version Date: 20151201

Printed and bound in India by Replika Press Pvt. Ltd.

International Standard Book Number-13: 978-1-4822-4450-2 (Pack - Book and Ebook)

Visit the Taylor & Francis Web site at
http://www.taylorandfrancis.com

and the CRC Press Web site at
http://www.crcpress.com

To those we teach
and from whom we learn:

Our fellows, residents, and medical students

EXECUTIVE EDITOR Sue Hodgson
SENIOR PROJECT EDITING MANAGER Carolyn Reich
SENIOR DEVELOPMENTAL EDITOR Megan Fennell
GRAPHICS MANAGER Brett Stone
DIRECTOR OF ILLUSTRATION AND DESIGN Brenda Bunch
BOOK DESIGN Jayne Jones
PROJECT MANAGER Kelly Mabie
MANUSCRIPT EDITOR Rebecca Sweeney
PRODUCTIONIST Debra Clark
PROOFREADER Linda Maulin
INDEXER Matthew White

Preface

Over the course of the past 15 years at our respective institutions—Washington University and Stanford University—we have had the honor and pleasure of training hundreds of medical students, residents (both orthopedic and plastic), and hand fellows. We have found that teaching hand surgery is best done while standing in front of a patient, while looking at a radiograph, or while settling in at the operating table. The education is personal and is focused on that specific hand problem.

The scope of hand and upper extremity surgery—from the shoulder to the fingertip and from skin to bone—can be overwhelming. However, we have realized that many themes repeat; the same hand problems present over and over. We decided that most of the core principles in hand surgery can be presented in 100 illustrative case examples. This book, *100 Hand Cases,* attempts to cover these key principles of hand surgery with straightforward treatment of classic hand problems.

This book will be an easy read. Only one photo per chapter is shown on purpose, and the presentation and treatment of each problem are concise. It is exactly what we discuss with our students, residents, and fellows in several focused minutes at the bedside or operating table. This book is designed for the learner to have an overview of the entire spectrum of hand surgery and to become familiar and comfortable with the most common hand problems. Key articles are listed for those who wish to delve deeper.

Special thanks to Julia Roeder Chang and Angela Sotelo for your wonderful transcription, editing, and organization.

We hope this book will give surgeons of every level confidence in treating the myriad clinical presentations that make up the extraordinary field of hand surgery.

Martin I. Boyer
James Chang

Contents

PART VIII   Dupuytren Contracture

PART IX   Fractures/Dislocations/Nonunions/Malunions

PART XVIII   Tumors

PART XIX   Vascular Conditions

PART

I

Amputations/
Fingertip Injuries

1 Replantation

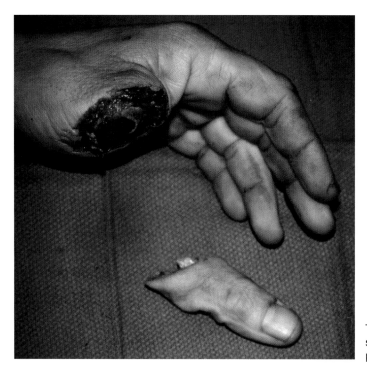

This 42-year-old construction worker has a saw injury to his left thumb, resulting in complete amputation.

Description of the Problem

The patient has a left thumb amputation. Because the thumb constitutes 40% of the function of the hand, referral to a tertiary hand center for emergent replantation is critical.

Key Anatomy

Replantation consists of complete reconstruction of all structures in the completely amputated part, whereas revascularization involves reestablishment of blood flow to the digit or part, but some portion of the part remains attached. In some cases, revascularization may be more difficult than replantation. In an amputated thumb, all of the component structures are completely transected, including the bones, joints, flexor tendons, extensor tendons, digital nerves, digital arteries, dorsal veins, and skin. Each structure needs to be carefully repaired to reestablish optimal function. In the thumb, the ulnar digital artery is almost three times larger than the radial digital artery. Therefore the ulnar digital artery is most suitable for microvascular anastomosis. However, this vessel is difficult to access with the hand in a supinated position.

Workup

Workup for any amputated part consists of careful screening for other associated emergent medical problems or conditions. A trauma workup is critical if there is evidence of any other injuries. The mechanism of the thumb amputation must be established. A patient with severe comorbidities may not be able to undergo such an extensive procedure. The patient is usually transferred from an outlying center as soon as possible to minimize ischemia time. The part is preserved in saline-moistened gauze placed in a plastic bag, which is placed in a container filled with ice water. This provides the most uniform cooling of the part while preventing direct contact with the ice. Radiographs of the hand and the thumb part are critical to assess for multilevel injuries. Patient consent is carefully obtained. Consent includes replantation; a possible bone graft, nerve graft, vein graft, and skin graft; possible joint fusion; and possible completion amputation. The patient should be carefully counseled that replantation is an unnatural act, but that all attempts will be undertaken to re-create the best possible function.

Treatment

The part is washed and prepared by isolating and identifying the digital nerves, the digital arteries, the dorsal veins, and the flexor and extensor tendons. The end of the bone is cleaned and sometimes shortened up to 1 cm to allow primary repair of the other structures. This dissection of the part can be performed while the patient is anesthetized. After the patient's hand is prepared and draped, the same structures are identified and tagged in the proximal hand. Small and medium clips are used to tag the digital vessels and digital nerves, respectively, so that they can be easily identified under the microscope later. In this specific case, the level of injury is at the metacarpophalangeal joint; therefore preparation for metacarpophalangeal joint fusion is essential. Because the ulnar digital artery is difficult to access, a vein is harvested from the wrist or foot and anastomosed to the amputated thumb part at the end of the ulnar digital artery. After this vein graft distal anastomosis is completed, the vein is carefully protected while bony fusion is performed. Using 90-90 intraosseous wire fixation allows good fixation of the metacarpophalangeal fusion without tethering the interphalangeal joint distally. The flexor tendon is repaired with a four-strand technique to facilitate early active motion. The extensor tendon is then repaired using a series of horizontal mattress sutures. With a tourniquet still inflated, the digital nerves are repaired under the microscope. We routinely then identify and repair the dorsal veins before deflating the tourniquet. We do this instead of the classic teaching of anastomosing the dorsal veins last, because it is easier to anastomose these veins while the field is blood free. Once the dorsal veins are anastomosed, the skin is reapproximated loosely on the dorsum, and the vein graft is brought proximally to the radial artery in the snuffbox. This vein graft is then anastomosed either end to side or end to end to the radial artery in the snuffbox. The hand is more easily positioned in this arrangement; therefore the proximal microvascular anastomosis of the artery to the vein graft is easier and less susceptible to technical failure. The vein graft is covered dorsally with an unmeshed split-thickness skin graft. A volar splint is placed, providing good access to the tip of the thumb. After thumb replantation, blood flow is easily evaluated with pulse oximetry.

Alternatives

There are specific indications and contraindications for replantation; however, the thumb must be replanted. Therefore all attempts at replantation must be made, including a referral to designated replantation centers. If the replantation is unsuccessful, then the patient may undergo elective thumb reconstruction at a later time.

Principles and Clinical Pearls

- A thumb replantation should always be attempted.
- Several "tricks," including performing the distal vein graft first and dorsal vein anastomoses before tourniquet deflation, have made thumb replantation easier and more reliable.
- A flexor tendon repair is the most important part of the operation, because it will determine the ultimate result of a digit that is likely to be replanted.

Pitfalls

Thumb replantation is a technically difficult procedure in inexperienced hands. The pitfalls include thumb ischemia after replantation, requiring microsurgical exploration; stiffness of the digit; and a poorly functioning digit. Attention to detail and patience are required at the initial replantation surgery.

Classic References

Chang J, Jones N. Twelve simple maneuvers to optimize digital replantation and revascularization. Tech Hand Up Extrem Surg 8:161, 2004.
This article showed twelve simple maneuvers to increase success rates for replantation and revascularization. It is a useful guide for those with experience performing replantation.

Jazayeri L, Klausner J, Chang J. Distal digital replantation. Plast Reconstr Surg 132:1207, 2013.
This paper specifically described indications and treatment algorithms for distal replantation; that is, at the level of the thumb interphalangeal joint or the finger distal interphalangeal joint. Specific tips and tricks in this article make distal digital replantation worthwhile.

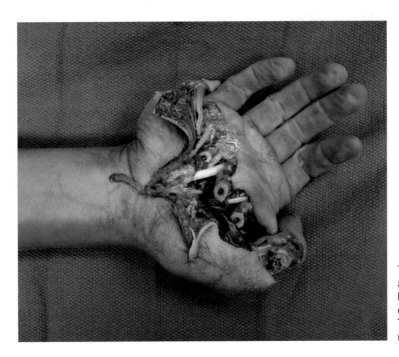

This 16-year-old boy has a hand near amputation from a rollover motor vehicle accident. The wound contained extensive dirt that has been debrided. The patient was taken to the operating room.

Description of the Problem

The patient has a hand near amputation at the level of the finger metacarpals and the thumb proximal phalanx. Bone, muscle, nerve, and vessel damage is extensive. The hand is devascularized. This will require immediate exploration and repair with further reconstruction in the future.

Key Anatomy

This operation requires an understanding of the detailed anatomy of the entire hand; specifically, the course of the median and ulnar nerves as they branch into common digital nerves is important. The contributions of the ulnar artery and radial artery to the superficial palmar arch and of the princeps pollicis artery to the thumb are critical for revascularization. Proper orientation of the flexor digitorum profundus and flexor digital superficialis tendons is necessary. The ulnar digital artery is much larger than the radial digital artery and is more favorable for microanastomosis and revascularization of the thumb.

Workup

As with any polytrauma case, a full trauma workup is essential. The cervical spine must be addressed. Once all life-threatening injuries are explored, attention can focus on the injured extremity. Radiographs are required to evaluate fractures and bone loss. The wound should not be explored in detail in the emergency department, because the patient would suffer unnecessarily. The need for an emergency operation is evident. Proper consent includes repair of all injured structures; possible vein, nerve, bone, and skin grafting; and the possibility of completion amputation.

Treatment

The surgery begins with irrigation and debridement of all dirt and the necrotic tissue. A carpal tunnel release is performed to ensure adequate cleansing of the wound and identification of the proximal end of nerves and vessels. The palm is then opened to expose all of the common digital nerves and arteries, which are presumed transected from the accident. The ulnar digital artery to the thumb is dissected free. The fractured bones and flexor tendons are identified. In this case the dorsum of the hand is intact; therefore veins do not need to be addressed.

After exploration and tagging of cut structures, bone fixation is performed using crossed K-wires for the metacarpals and the thumb proximal phalanx. Plates are not used because of the contaminated wound. The flexor tendons are repaired in zone III using a multistrand repair. While the tourniquet is inflated, the common digital nerves are repaired or grafted using the operating microscope. The ulnar motor nerve and the median motor branch to the thumb are repaired as necessary.

The tourniquet is deflated, and proximal arterial inflow is confirmed. Vein grafts from the foot are harvested to provide conduits from the proximal arteries to the distal vessels. Given the mechanism of the accident, loss of vessels is possible. The microanatomoses need to be performed outside of the zone of injury; therefore vein grafts are required. The skin is then closed, with skin grafting as necessary.

Alternatives

This is an acutely devascularized hand. There are no alternatives other than immediate operative exploration and microvascular repair. Failure to attempt this will surely lead to amputation and loss of hand function.

Principles and Clinical Pearls
- Immediate exploration and debridement are critical.
- The specific sequence of repair—bones, tendons, nerves, and arteries—allows most of the operation to be performed in a bloodless field.
- Vein grafting out of the zone of injury will prevent thrombosis.

Pitfalls
This is a very difficult operation. The pitfalls include devascularization, skin loss, and stiffness. Revision surgery for tendon adhesions and/or contracture release may be necessary.

Classic References

Chang J, Jones N. Twelve simple maneuvers to optimize digital replantation. Tech Hand Up Extrem Surg 8:161, 2004.
This technique paper highlighted tips and tricks to facilitate replantation.

Paavilainen P, Nietosvaara Y, Tikkinen KA, Salmi T, Paakkala T, Vilkki S. Long-term results of transmetacarpal replantation. J Plast Reconstr Aesthet Surg 60:704, 2007.
This was a very large retrospective review of transmetacarpal revascularization and replantation cases. There were amazingly 43 patients in this series. The authors concluded that this was a favorable zone of injury, with most transmetacarpal injuries revascularized or replanted resulting in good subjective and satisfactory functional results.

3 Mutilated Arm Injury

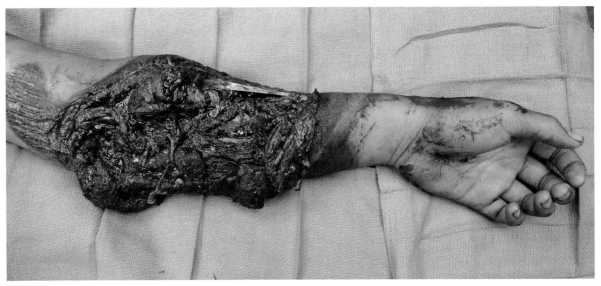

This patient is seen in the emergency department after a rollover motor vehicle accident. The patient's left arm was outside the driver's seat window as the car rolled. He was stabilized in the field and transferred in a helicopter.

Description of the Problem

The patient has a severe mutilating injury of the left upper extremity. Skin and muscle loss is significant, with probable nerve and vessel injury and underlying fractures. The arm may be devascularized. The wound is contaminated and will require emergent exploration, debridement, and repair.

Key Anatomy

Knowledge of the entire anatomy of the upper extremity is essential to reconstruct this arm. Particular attention is paid to nerve pathways, flexor and extensor tendon function, and the vascular supply for flap coverage.

Workup

This is a major traumatic injury in a patient with life-threatening injuries. The patient requires assessment and stabilization in the trauma unit. The cervical spine status must be evaluated. A full trauma workup is performed, beginning with the ABCs—airway, breathing, and circulation. Trauma surgeons must clear the patient for surgery.

A preoperative evaluation includes assessment of the vascular status and the neuromuscular status. Probing of the wound is not necessary, because the patient will need definitive intraoperative debridement. Radiographs of the hand, forearm, and elbow are critical. If the patient has no palpable pulses, capillary refill, and/or Doppler signal, then angiography will be necessary to assess the vascular status. The patient should be counseled on the need for multiple operative procedures, the possible need for flaps and grafts, and the possible need for arm amputation in the future.

Treatment

The operation begins with irrigation and radical debridement. All contaminated and devitalized tissue is removed. In this case, a significant amount of muscle must be debrided. The skin and fascia are opened to prevent compartment syndrome. A carpal tunnel release is performed as part of the compartment release and to localize the median nerve. Any fractures are treated with external fixation because of the contaminated wound. If the wound is well cleaned, nerve and tendon repairs are performed if they can be done primarily. The wound is dressed and a second look is scheduled for 24 to 48 hours later. On second look, any remaining devitalized tissue is removed. Definitive tendon and nerve repairs are done, including grafting as necessary. The soft tissue coverage is planned. Given the extensive nature of this injury, a free tissue transfer is likely. In this case, a large muscle flap such as the latissimus dorsi muscle flap or a fasciocutaneous flap such as an anterolateral thigh flap will be required. The flap is performed only after the wound is clean. Inflow and outflow vessels are carefully chosen to prevent devascularizing the hand. The flap procedure should account for the need for delayed tendon, bone, or nerve reconstruction once the wound is covered.

Alternatives

There are many alternatives for every choice of tendon, bone, and nerve reconstruction and flap reconstruction, depending on the tissues that require debridement. The major alternative in this case is arm amputation; however, given the intact hand distally, all efforts should be made in limb salvage.

Principles and Clinical Pearls

- Radical debridement is performed until all devitalized tissue is removed.
- Fractures are stabilized with minimal internal hardware.
- Early nerve and tendon reconstruction is performed once the wound is clean.
- The goal of all decision-making, including flap coverage, is to maximize function and the aesthetic appearance of the arm.

Pitfalls

In this complex case, pitfalls arise at every step. The main preventable problems include (1) inadequate debridement leading to infection, (2) a poorly designed and executed free tissue transfer leading to flap loss, and (3) missed compartment syndrome.

Classic Reference

Hsu CC, Lin YT, Lin CH, Lin CH, Wei FC. Immediate emergency free anterolateral thigh flap transfer for the mutilated upper extremity. Plast Reconstr Surg 123:1739, 2009.

Much of the literature in mutilated arm injuries exist in book chapters, because the techniques are standard and outcomes studies are few. However, this study highlighted the use of the anterolateral thigh flap. This is a versatile, large flap that can be harvested from an uninvolved limb by a second team.

4 Thumb Pulp Defect

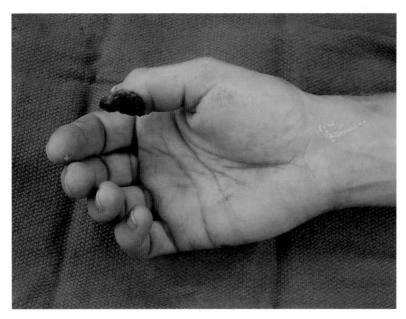

This patient has a degloving injury of her right thumb pulp.

Description of the Problem

The patient has near-complete loss of the entire thumb pulp. The dorsal extensor apparatus and nail are intact. The distal phalanx bone and flexor tendon are exposed.

Key Anatomy

The thumb pulp is a critical area, because so much of the hand function is based on the thumb. The thumb pulp provides fine sensation and covers the underlying flexor pollicis longus tendon and distal phalanx. At the level of the thumb interphalangeal joint, the digital nerves trifurcate and branch to provide sensation throughout the entire thumb pulp.

Workup

As in any hand trauma patient, radiographs are critical to assess for an underlying fracture or dislocation. Although the thumb pulp is missing, the patient should be tested for extension and flexion of the thumb. The exposed bone and flexor tendon are visualized. A dressing should be applied to cover the wound until definitive coverage is performed.

Treatment

Coverage of the thumb pulp is critical to restore function to the hand. The thumb should not be shortened. Therefore treatment involving only removal of the exposed bone and closure of the thumb pulp are discouraged. Instead, adequate flap coverage with sensation is preferred. A skin graft is not useful in this situation, because it would provide minimal sensation and the thumb pulp would be flat. Several options for sensory soft tissue coverage are available. The simplest flap option is a cross-finger flap from the dorsum of the index finger. The dorsal digital nerve can be coapted to the ulnar digital nerve to the thumb. However, this requires a period of immobilization of the hand and separation of the cross-finger flap several weeks later. A preferred alternative is the first dorsal metacarpal artery flap. The flap is designed over the dorsum of the proximal phalanx to the index finger. The first dorsal metacarpal artery is traced back along with the dorsal digital nerve and then transposed to cover the thumb pulp by tunneling underneath the proximal thumb skin. In this case, the dorsal digital nerve can be coapted to the ulnar digital nerve to provide better sensation. This is a one-stage procedure, compared with a cross-finger flap. A third alternative is a free toe pulp flap; however, this requires microsurgical anastomosis.

Alternatives

A preferred flap is the first dorsal metacarpal artery flap. A cross-finger flap and a free toe pulp flap are excellent alternatives. Surgeons should be dissuaded from shortening the bone or placing skin graft as a cover.

Principles and Clinical Pearls

- Hand surgeons should understand the importance of the thumb pulp in providing sensation and bulk.
- A first dorsal metacarpal artery flap is a very versatile and reliable flap for thumb pulp coverage.
- The thumb length should be maintained at all costs to provide optimal function.

Pitfalls

Pitfalls include flap loss of the first dorsal metacarpal artery flap. This flap should be carefully designed, and care should be taken to preserve the vascular pedicle. If the flap is unsuccessful, the alternatives described previously are available.

Classic References

Chen C, Zhang X, Shao X, Gao S, Wang B, Liu D. Treatment of thumb tip degloving injury using the modified first dorsal metacarpal artery flap. J Hand Surg Am 35:1663, 2010.
The first dorsal metacarpal artery flap was designed with dorsal nerves to restore sensation to the tip of the thumb.

Germann G, Sauerbier M, Rudolf KD, Hrabowski M. Management of thumb tip injuries. J Hand Surg Am 40:614, 2015.
This was an excellent review of the management of thumb tip injuries. The authors reviewed the entire algorithm for thumb pulp flap coverage, including semiocclusive dressings as a simple and inexpensive alternative.

5 Fingertip Defect

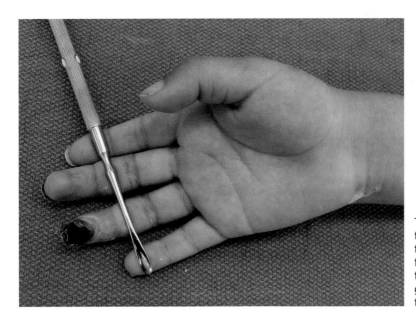

This 12-year-old girl is seen in consultation. She has a soft tissue defect of the tip of her right ring finger. Her ring finger was caught in a car door, and the piece was replaced in the emergency department. Now, 5 days after the accident, the skin has necrosed.

Description of the Problem

The patient has a full-thickness loss of most of the distal pad of the right ring finger. Soft tissue bulk and sensation to the tip are missing. Once the necrotic tissue is debrided, the distal phalanx bone will be exposed. The nail on the dorsum is intact.

Key Anatomy

At the level of the distal interphalangeal joint, the digital artery and nerve begin to trifurcate into terminal branches. The volar skin protects the underlying distal phalanx bone. Sensation is critical for fine touch and manipulation. Therefore sensation, soft tissue cover, and fingertip bulk need to be restored for optimal reconstruction.

Workup

The wound is evaluated in the clinic, but the tissue defect is thoroughly assessed intraoperatively after debridement. Radiographs are critical to rule out distal phalanx dislocation or fracture. The rest of the hand, including the adjacent fingers, is carefully evaluated for evidence of prior trauma and wounds. This is done to assess donor sites for various local and pedicled flap options.

Treatment

The wound is debrided thoroughly. In this case, reconstruction will require full-thickness skin and soft tissue. Sensate skin would be optimal. Our choice for reconstruction is an innervated cross-finger flap from the dorsum of the middle finger. The skin over the middle phalanx dorsum is raised with the skin bridge on the radial side. Care is taken to raise the skin in a full-thickness fashion, leaving the paratenon of the extensor tendon in place for later skin grafting. The dorsal digital nerve is identified and dissected proximally. The nerve is transected proximal to where it enters the flap. Along the radial base, Cleland ligaments should be released to prevent kinking of the skin flap on inset. The flap is positioned onto the volar side of the index finger wound. The flap should be tension free. Before skin closure, the dorsal digital nerve in the flap is coapted to one of the cut digital nerves in the index finger to restore some degree of sensation. The flap is sewn in place, and the donor site on the middle finger dorsum is covered with a full-thickness skin graft. The hand is then splinted in a comfortable position. Three weeks later, the fingers are divided and range of motion movement is begun.

Alternatives

For small fingertip wounds, healing by secondary intention can be effective. Wounds smaller than 1 cm² may heal with daily dressing changes. However, this is unlikely to be as effective in healing the entire distal pulp. Skin grafts are not used, because they would not replace the bulk and sensation of the finger pad. Other viable flap options include a reverse homodigital island flap and a thenar flap.

Principles and Clinical Pearls

- If the entire finger volar pad is missing, replacement of skin cover, tissue bulk, and sensation is essential.
- Hand surgeons should be comfortable performing a cross-finger flap, because it is a workhorse intrinsic flap in the hand.
- An innervated cross-finger flap is a simple variation and may increase sensation in this important contact area.

Pitfalls

Flap loss, skin graft loss, and dehiscence are the preventable complications. The flap is circular and may form a "biscuitlike" appearance because of the circumferential scar line. This can be corrected with Z-plasties. Flexion contracture is not likely if aggressive range of motion exercises are performed immediately after flap division.

Classic References

Lee NH, Pae WS, Roh SG, Oh KJ, Bae CS, Yang KM. Innervated cross-finger pulp flap for reconstruction of the fingertip. Arch Plast Surg 39:637, 2012.
In this series from Korea, the authors presented their technique on variations of the innervated cross-finger flaps. Their experience was large, with 69 cases.

Matsui J, Piper S, Boyer M. Nonmicrosurgical options for soft tissue reconstruction of the hand. Curr Rev Musculoskelet Med 7:68, 2014.
This was an excellent review of all nonmicrosurgical techniques for soft tissue reconstruction of the hand. The options ranged from healing by secondary intention and local care to skin grafting and to the classic intrinsic flaps to the hand. The authors showed that several options may exist for each type of wound. Surgery should be tailored to the patient.

Tang JB, Eliot D, Adani R, Saint-Cyr M, Stang F. Repair and reconstruction of thumb and finger tip injuries: a global view. Clin Plast Surg 41:325, 2014.
This was a very fun paper to read. The premise is that flap choice for finger reconstruction differs worldwide. Experts from around the world listed their flap of choice for specific defects. Alternatively, there were many viable flap options for each defect. Many excellent pictures show the operative technique.

6 Total Thumb Reconstruction

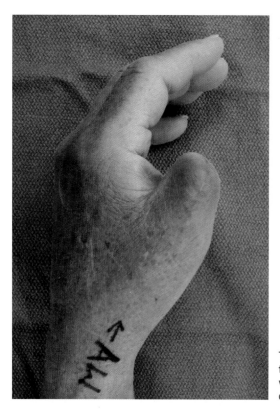

This 22-year-old laborer has a crush avulsion injury to his left thumb. The thumb was not replantable at the time of injury. The wound was closed, and the patient now returns requesting reconstruction.

Description of the Problem

The patient has a total thumb amputation requiring reconstruction to restore acceptable hand function. The radiographs show that the amputation is just distal to the metacarpophalangeal joint. At this level, the patient will have difficulty using his thumb to pinch and grasp larger objects. He may be concerned with the aesthetic appearance of this shortened thumb. Most patients with a thumb amputation at this level will request reconstruction.

Key Anatomy

The level of thumb amputation is critical to determining the best treatment. An amputation of the distal tip usually only requires some soft tissue coverage but not bone reconstruction. Patients whose amputation is at the level of the interphalangeal joint may or may not request reconstruction, because length is usually sufficient to provide some pinch activity. In patients whose amputation is more proximal at the level of the proximal phalanx or metacarpophalangeal joint, the length is typically too short for adequate daily use. Amputations at this level require complex reconstruction with either a toe-to-thumb transfer or an osteoplastic reconstruction. If the amputation is at the level of the proximal metacarpal, then even more complex reconstruction requiring a bone graft and toe-to-thumb transfer may be required in a staged fashion. If the thenar muscles and carpometacarpal joint have been obliterated by the accident, then an index pollicization should be considered as an alternative approach.

Workup

The nature of the injury must be reviewed for evidence of more proximal tissue injury. In this case, the amputation is limited to the distal thumb. Radiographs of the hand and ipsilateral foot should be obtained in preparation for a great toe-to-thumb transfer. If a proximal injury in the hand and wrist is evident, then an angiogram may be necessary. The target vessel for revascularization of the toe-to-thumb transfer is the radial artery in the dorsal snuffbox; therefore adequate flow through the ulnar artery must be confirmed.

Treatment

This patient underwent treatment with a great toe-to-thumb transfer. This was performed in a staged fashion. To limit the skin defect on the donor foot, the patient first underwent a groin flap to allow a sleeve of skin on the remaining hand to be fashioned. After several months, the second-stage operation was completed with a great toe-to-thumb transfer. The flexor hallucis longus tendon in a great toe was tunneled into the distal forearm and transferred to the flexor digitorum superficialis tendon to the ring finger to provide a new motor for thumb flexion. The extensor hallucis longus tendon was repaired to the extensor pollicis longus tendon proximally. The first dorsal metatarsal artery was anastomosed to the radial artery, and the dorsal veins were anastomosed to their respective veins in the hand. The digital nerves were coapted to provide sensation. In many instances, the anastomosis would be too tight by directly closing the wound; therefore a skin graft is placed over the dorsum of the hand.

Alternatives

There are several alternatives to a great toe-to-thumb transfer. One is a trimmed great toe in which the lateral third of the toe is excised and the nail fold reconstructed to allow transfer of a thinner toe. This can be done either at the time of toe transfer or, as we prefer, in a delayed fashion. Other toe-to-thumb transfer alternatives include a great-toe wraparound flap and a second-toe transfer. A great-toe wraparound flap does not allow interphalangeal joint flexion, and a transferred second toe does not mimic the shape and form of the thumb as well as a great toe.

Principles and Clinical Pearls

- The length of the thumb defect determines the optimal reconstructive option.
- A groin flap is necessary in many instances to provide a sleeve of skin, thus minimizing skin that is removed from the foot.
- Careful microsurgical technique is critical to ensure the toe is successful.

Pitfalls

Complications in this operation include poor function after toe transfer and failure of the toe. The tendon and nerve repairs require great care to ensure optimal function. A classic mistake is to be short of skin; therefore a groin flap is frequently necessary, especially to resurface the thumb-index web space and for dorsal skin coverage.

Classic References

Waljee JF, Chung KC. Toe-to-hand transfer: evolving indications and relevant outcomes. J Hand Surg Am 38:1431, 2013.
This focused review highlighted the indications and the various drawbacks of each procedure.

Wei FC, Chen HC, Chuang CC, Chen SH. Microsurgical thumb reconstruction with toe transfer: selection of various techniques. Plast Reconstr Surg 93:345, 1994.
This truly classic article discussed the various options for toe transfer. The Chang Gung group had the largest experience in toe transfer in the world.

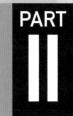

PART

II

Anesthesia and Pain Management

7 Complex Regional Pain Syndrome

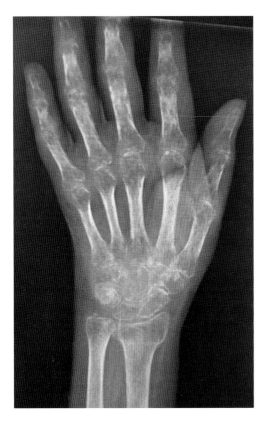

This 38-year-old woman presents with a 4-month history of pain, stiffness, decreased strength, and an inability to return to work after experiencing a minor work-related injury in which her hand and wrist were caught between a sliding glass steel door and its frame. She has no abrasions or external signs of trauma, and plain radiographs are negative. At the time of injury, a physical examination revealed diffuse tenderness on palpation of the dorsal carpus. A physical examination on presentation to the office reveals a bright glassy complexion to the skin, passive and active digital stiffness in attempted flexion, diffuse tenderness on palpation of the dorsal and volar carpus, and decreased objective two-point discrimination in the median nerve distribution.

Description of the Problem

Subacute, nonspecific signs and symptoms consisting of pain, tenderness, digital stiffness, and skin discoloration and tightness are highly suggestive of complex regional pain syndrome type 1 (CRSP1). The diagnosis is one of exclusion—bony, ligamentous, and tendon injuries should be ruled out by clinical examination and appropriate imaging; peripheral nerve injury and compression syndromes should be ruled out by clinical examination and electrophysiologic assessment; and vascular injury should be ruled out by clinical examination and either non-invasive or invasive studies, as indicated. Once a correctable cause has been ruled out, CRPS1 can be diagnosed. A three-phase bone scan has been used historically for diagnosis, but presently its usefulness is open to debate. A differential diagnosis includes carpal tunnel compression of the median nerve (see Chapters 21 and 68), radial sensory nerve neuritis (see Chapter 8), lateral antebrachial sensory nerve neuritis, Guyon canal compression of the ulnar nerve (see Chapter 70), ulnar or radial artery injury, and injury to the metacarpus, the carpus, or the distal radius and ulna. Tendinosis or tendinitis of the first dorsal compartment, the sixth dorsal compartment, and the flexor carpi radialis should be considered. A diagnosis is based on a clinical examination and the observation of diffuse osteopenia on plain radiographs, with normal vascular and electrophysiologic assessments. An MRI of the affected area can be useful to rule out structural lesions.

Key Anatomy

Patients are evaluated for point tenderness and signs of peripheral nerve compression or irritation in all the usual anatomic locations.

Workup

Imaging studies include plain radiographs of the hand and wrist, electrophysiologic assessment, MRI (optional), three-phase bone scan (optional), and vascular studies (optional).

Treatment

The initial treatment should focus on evaluation and treatment of any structural lesion causing the pain syndrome to persist. Most frequently, this consists of relieving compression of the median nerve in the carpal tunnel (thus a diagnosis of CRPS2 is appropriate) by a carpal tunnel release. Other modalities such as sympathetic ganglion (stellate ganglion) blocks, oral medications (gabapentin and antidepressants) can be attempted. The stiff digits and thumb can be mobilized while the patient is anesthetized.

Alternatives

There are no alternative treatments.

Principles and Clinical Pearls

- A careful physical examination is essential to evaluate for a structural lesion that might be correctable by surgery. The most commonly encountered phenomenon in these cases is median nerve compression in the carpal tunnel. The signs and symptoms of carpal tunnel syndrome in these patients may be subtle, and the electrical studies may be read as *normal*. This should not dissuade a treating surgeon from active treatment of the median nerve compression.
- These patients should not be given long-term oral narcotic medications.

Pitfalls

The main difficulty in treating patients who have CRPS1 is to rule out significant psychological effects that exacerbate the patient's complaints and to rule out a structural lesion that might benefit from a surgical remedy. Long-term oral medication may be helpful in some cases, but rarely if ever do these medications include narcotics.

Classic Reference

Placzek JD, Boyer MI, Gelberman RH, Sopp B, Goldfarb CA. Nerve decompression for complex regional pain syndrome type II following upper extremity surgery. J Hand Surg Am 30:69, 2005.
In the setting of either clinical or electrophysiologic evidence of peripheral nerve compression, surgical treatment may hasten recovery in patients with CRPS2.

8 Radial Sensory Neuritis

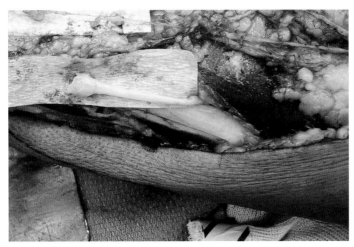

This 28-year-old business manager has a degloving laceration to his left forearm caused by a motor vehicle accident. Because of the severity of his other injuries, the wound was not explored at the time of his initial presentation. Six months later, he continued to have lancinating pain radiating toward the dorsal aspect of the thumb-index web space, and hypesthesia was noted on physical examination in the area. A Tinel sign was elicited on percussion of the area. Plain radiographs showed no abnormalities.

Description of the Problem

Radial sensory neuritis can be traumatic in origin (as in this case) or caused by an idiopathic compression of the radial nerve by the tendon of the brachioradialis (Wartenberg syndrome). In some patients, the symptoms are preceded or exacerbated by twisting motions. A differential diagnosis includes de Quervain tendinitis or tenosynovitis (see Chapter 81), intersection syndrome, lateral antebrachial cutaneous nerve (LABCN) neuritis or injury, C6 radiculopathy, a proximal radial nerve injury or neuritis, and a radial fracture (see Chapters 41 and 42).

Key Anatomy

The sensory branch of the radial nerve emerges from deep to the brachioradialis approximately 6 cm proximal to the radial styloid process and is prone to injury or compression in this area. The terminal branch of the musculocutaneous nerve (LABCN) innervates the skin over the basal joint of the thumb and the proximal aspect of the thenar eminence, and travels superficial to the cephalic vein, whereas the radial nerve travels deep to it. The radial sensory nerve innervates the skin over the dorsum of the thumb, the index and middle fingers, and the skin overlying the first dorsal interosseous muscle. The intersection between the first (abductor pollicis longus and extensor pollicis brevis) and second (extensor carpi radialis longus and extensor carpi radialis brevis) compartments are subjacent to the nerve. A terminal branch of the radial sensory nerve lies directly on the tendon of the extensor pollicis longus, over the thumb metacarpal. This branch is at risk of iatrogenic injury in dorsal approaches to the distal radius on release of the third dorsal compartment and in radiodorsal approaches to the ulnar collateral ligament of the thumb metacarpophalangeal joint.

Workup

An electrophysiologic assessment is unreliable in the diagnosis of this condition. Plain radiographs are useful to rule out associated bony injury, and an MRI may help to rule out associated soft tissue injury or tendinitis.

Treatment

For Wartenberg syndrome, splinting of the wrist and thumb should be attempted. A corticosteroid with or without a local anesthetic can be injected directly into the area of the maximal Tinel sign. These injections can be repeated as necessary. Operative treatment consists of decompression of the point of emergence of the nerve from under the brachioradialis. If the nerve has been lacerated and a neuroma has developed, then treatment consists of excising the neuroma and either performing a nerve graft or burying the nerve end into muscle or bone.

Alternatives

Concurrent C6 radiculopathy should be sought. Cervical spine range of motion should be tested. Patients should be evaluated for the presence of a Spurling sign and weakness of the wrist extensor muscles.

Principles and Clinical Pearls

- Classic Wartenberg syndrome (cheiralgia paresthetica) is the eponym given to compression of the sensory branch of the radial nerve in this area.
- Surgical treatment of Wartenberg syndrome is rarely required.
- If a traumatic neuroma is present, then a nerve graft is performed or the nerve end is buried into muscle or bone.
- If surgery is performed, the risk of iatrogenic nerve injury is minimized by identifying the nerve deep to the tendon of the brachioradialis, proximal to the site of compression.

Pitfalls

Complications of treatment include persistence of sensory disturbance and pain and recurrence.

Classic Reference

Braidwood AS. Superficial radial neuropathy. J Bone Joint Surg Br 57:380, 1975.
The authors included anatomy in their description of a series of 12 patients, 6 of whom improved with nonoperative measures and two of whom improved with local injections of hydrocortisone.

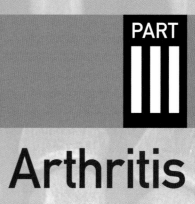

Arthritis

9 Thumb Carpometacarpal Joint Osteoarthritis

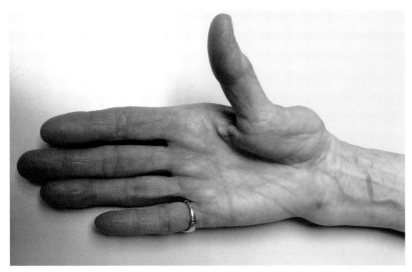

This 70-year-old woman has a 1-year history of steadily increasing pain in her right hand when unscrewing lids off of jars, turning keys in locks, gripping and rotating doorknobs, holding a pen, and pinching her grandchildren's cheeks. A physical examination reveals tenderness over the thumb carpometacarpal (CMC) joint dorsally. Passive adduction of the thumb CMC joint reproduces the pain.

Description of the Problem

Trapeziometacarpal osteoarthritis (CMC osteoarthritis) involves progressive loss of articular cartilage on the proximal aspect of the thumb metacarpal and the distal trapezium. This is thought to be associated with attenuation of the so-called beak ligament (the volar oblique ligament of the CMC joint), in which the metacarpal base subluxes dorsally and migrates proximally. The CMC joint often becomes stiff, and thumb hyperextension occurs at the metacarpophalangeal (MCP) joint. This causes progressive laxity of the MCP joint from volar plate and ulnar collateral ligament attenuation. A differential diagnosis includes scaphotrapeziotrapezoid osteoarthritis (see Chapter 10), de Quervain tenosynovitis (see Chapter 81), radial sensory nerve irritation (Wartenberg syndrome) (see Chapter 8), scaphoid fracture or nonunion (see Chapters 50 and 51), and radioscaphoid osteoarthritis.

Key Anatomy

The thumb CMC joint is a saddle-shaped articulation, allowing motion in flexion-extension, abduction-adduction, and rotational directions. It is stabilized statically by its capsule and intracapsular ligaments (of which the anterior oblique ligament and the intermetacarpal ligament are the two most critical) and has little or no intrinsic bony stability. The trapezium articulates with the thumb metacarpal distally and with the distal scaphoid, the proximal-radial second metacarpal, and the radial trapezoid proximally. The dorsal approach to the thumb CMC joint introduces the deep branch of the radial artery into the operative field. The volar (Wagner) approach involves terminal branches of the lateral antebrachial cutaneous nerve and the sensory branch of the radial nerve.

Workup

PA, lateral, and hyperpronated plain radiographs of the thumb base provide the best visualization of the CMC joint. The presence or absence of scaphotrapezial osteoarthritis should be noted.

Treatment

Treatment options include activity modification, a forearm-based or hand-based splint (either custom-molded or off-the-shelf), oral antiinflammatory agents given on a scheduled basis, and/or intraarticular injections of a corticosteroid with or without a local anesthetic. Injections can be repeated as necessary. Operative treatment involves either trapezial excision or hemiexcision with or without ligament reconstruction (using tendons from the abductor pollicis longus, the flexor carpi radialis, or the extensor carpi radialis longus) of the thumb CMC joint. These procedures require 6 weeks of immobilization postoperatively, followed by an additional 6 to 10 weeks of therapy to improve anteposition and strength. Concurrent arthritis and hyperextension of the MCP joint of the thumb may require capsulodesis or arthrodesis.

Alternatives

Arthrodesis of the thumb CMC joint is an alternative for patients who want a strong, stable grip. Some surgeons have advocated metacarpal extension osteotomy or implant arthroplasty; however, these have not gained wide-spread acceptance.

Principles and Clinical Pearls

- In the absence of clinically relevant scaphotrapeziotrapezoid osteoarthritis, CMC fusion may be considered in younger, more active patients, and CMC arthroplasty (with or without ligament reconstruction) may be reserved for older, less active patients.
- Forty percent of patients with early thumb CMC osteoarthritis have up to 18 months (or longer) of relief after intraarticular injection of corticosteroids.
- Thumb MCP arthrodesis may be performed concurrently with thumb CMC excision arthroplasty if pain and instability are present at the MCP joint.

Pitfalls

The many pitfalls include infection, nonunion (for arthrodesis) wound dehiscence, radial sensory nerve irritation or injury, lateral antebrachial cutaneous nerve irritation or injury, proximal metacarpal subsidence, proximal metacarpal adduction, weakness, incomplete pain relief, and underappreciated scaphotrapezoid osteoarthritis.

Classic Reference

Eaton RG, Lane LB, Littler JW, Keyser JJ. Ligament reconstruction for the painful thumb carpometacarpal joint: a long-term assessment. J Hand Surg Am 9:692, 1984.
This classic article described ligament reconstruction without tendon interposition for the treatment of early thumb CMC arthritis. Although the article advocated the use of this operation once arthritis was visible on plain radiographs, most surgeons would resect the trapeziometacarpal joint in these cases and then reconstruct the thumb base using the flexor carpi radialis or the abductor pollicis longus tendon.

10 Scaphotrapeziotrapezoid Joint Osteoarthritis

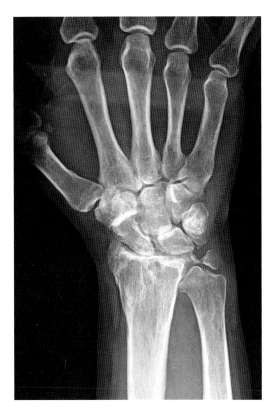

This 43-year-old male steel worker has a 2-year history of progressive pain in his radial wrist and weakness of grip and pinch. He has no history of trauma. A physical examination reveals tenderness to palpation in the anatomic snuffbox.

Description of the Problem

The patient has decreased articular cartilage between the proximal aspects of the trapezium and trapezoid bones and the distal pole of the scaphoid. Scaphotrapeziotrapezoid (STT) osteoarthritis is much less common than thumb carpometacarpal (CMC) osteoarthritis as an isolated condition. It occurs in younger patients and is more resistant to nonoperative treatment. A differential diagnosis includes thumb CMC arthritis (see Chapter 9), de Quervain tenosynovitis (see Chapter 81), radial sensory nerve irritation (Wartenberg syndrome) (see Chapter 8), scaphoid fracture or nonunion (see Chapters 50 and 51), and radioscaphoid osteoarthritis. The diagnosis is based on the clinical examination and plain radiographic confirmation.

Key Anatomy

A direct surgical approach to the STT joint involves isolation of the deep branch of the radial artery in the anatomic snuffbox. The main blood supply to the scaphoid enters dorsally just proximal to the capsule insertion of the STT joint on the scaphoid. The extensor carpi radialis longus tendon inserts radially on the base of the index metacarpal and borders the operative field ulnarly, along with the extensor pollicis longus tendon. Radial styloid excision can improve visualization of the STT joint and facilitate harvest of a bone graft to enhance arthrodesis.

Workup

PA, lateral, and hyperpronated plain radiographs of the thumb base will show the STT joint.

Treatment

Treatment options include activity modification, a forearm-based splint (either custom-molded or off-the-shelf), oral antiinflammatory agents given on a scheduled basis, and/or fluoroscopy-assisted intraarticular injection of a corticosteroid with or without a local anesthetic. Injections can be repeated as necessary. Injection of hyaluronate has not been shown to be of significant benefit. In patients without thumb CMC osteoarthritis, STT arthrodesis is preferred. If clinically relevant thumb CMC disease is present with STT osteoarthritis, then complete trapeziectomy either with or without ligament reconstruction of the thumb CMC joint can be performed (using tendons from the abductor pollicis longus, the flexor carpi radialis, or the extensor carpi radialis longus). Both procedures require 6 weeks of immobilization postoperatively, followed by an additional 6 to 10 weeks of therapy to improve anteposition and strength. Full strength should not be expected until up to 2 years postoperatively. Occasionally, a CT scan of the STT joint may be required to confirm bony union.

Alternatives

Arthrodesis and arthroplasty are the only two surgical treatments currently.

Principles and Clinical Pearls

- A radial styloid excision helps substantially with exposure.
- Bone graft is used to pack the defect that is present after excision of the articular cartilage and subchondral bone.
- Fixation of the arthrodesis is challenging and can involve circular fixation, screws, K-wires, or bone staples.
- Arthrodesis is confirmed by progressive plain radiographic opacification of the STT joint and possibly an orthogonal CT scan.

Pitfalls

Complications of surgical arthrodesis include nonunion, infection, wound dehiscence, radial sensory nerve irritation or injury, lateral antebrachial cutaneous nerve irritation or injury, and incomplete pain relief. Radial artery injury can occur; a preoperative Allen test to demonstrate the ulnar arterial supply to the thumb and radial hand should be performed.

Classic Reference

Srinivasan VB, Matthews JP. Results of scaphotrapeziotrapezoid fusion for isolated idiopathic arthritis. J Hand Surg Br 21:378, 1996.
Seven of eight patients had successful arthrodesis and excellent or good pain relief, whereas the patient with a poor result had nonunion of the arthrodesis with persistent pain.

11 Metacarpophalangeal Joint Osteoarthritis

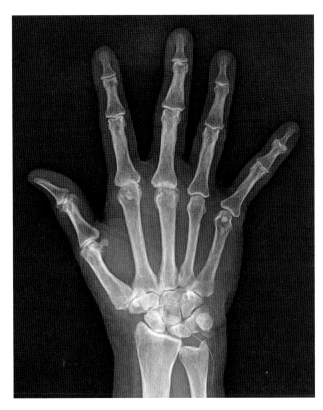

This 48-year-old male gravedigger has a 1-year history of progressive pain and loss of motion in the metacarpophalangeal (MCP) joint of his nondominant middle finger. A physical examination reveals tenderness to palpation at the volar and dorsal aspects of the MCP joint and limited range of motion of 15 to 55 degrees of flexion. Swelling is noticeable dorsally and in the dorsal aspect of the index-middle and the middle-ring interspaces, but no bruising or discrete mass is present.

Description of the Problem

The patient has decreased articular cartilage between the proximal aspect of the proximal phalanx and the metacarpal head. Often in patients with MCP joint osteoarthritis, a prominent dorsal osteophyte is present on the metacarpal and the proximal aspect of the articular surface of the metacarpal. Range of motion is limited frequently, and grip is weak. A differential diagnosis includes trigger finger (see Chapter 80). MCP joint osteoarthritis can be associated with systemic diseases such as hemochromatosis, rheumatoid arthritis, gout, and pseudogout.

Key Anatomy

The MCP joint is best accessed through a dorsal approach around the extensor tendon and a dorsal capsulectomy of the MCP joint.

Workup

PA, lateral, oblique, and Brewerton (20-degree MCP flexion PA view) plain radiographs of the MCP joint are needed. The presence of a joint effusion may indicate joint aspiration is necessary, with examination of the aspirate for crystals.

Treatment

Initial treatment includes activity modification, splint immobilization, oral antiinflammatory agents given on a scheduled basis, and/or intraarticular injection of a corticosteroid with or without a local anesthetic. Injections can be repeated as necessary. Injection of hyaluronate has not been shown to be of significant benefit. The FDA recently approved topical antiinflammatory agents such as diclofenac. Operative treatment can involve either MCP joint arthrodesis or MCP arthroplasty (with a silicone or metal and polyethylene prosthesis). Arthrodesis reliably relieves pain; however, motion loss at the MCP joint may be problematic, especially if concomitant PIP joint arthritis is present. Arthroplasty can be of benefit for pain relief but should not be relied on to improve range of motion.

Alternatives

Arthrodesis or arthroplasty are the only two surgical treatments currently. Interposition arthroplasty with a volar plate or other biologic tissues have been tried, but have not gained widespread acceptance.

Principles and Clinical Pearls

- Trigger finger is the main differential diagnosis. After injection for trigger finger without substantial relief of symptoms, MCP arthritis is often diagnosed radiographically. A dorsal injection of a corticosteroid can be given.
- Arthrodesis often requires the use of bone graft, because the presence of intact deep transverse metacarpal ligaments makes it difficult surgically to translate the proximal phalanx sufficiently proximal for direct bone-to-bone contact.

Pitfalls

Complications of surgical arthrodesis include nonunion, infection, and wound dehiscence. Complications of arthroplasty include implant loosening, implant breakage, joint instability (with excessive release of the MCP collateral ligament or ligaments), infection, and wound dehiscence. Patient expectations regarding range of motion postoperatively should be tempered.

Classic Reference

Feldon P, Belsky MR. Degenerative disease of the metacarpophalangeal joints. Hand Clin 3:429, 1987.
The authors reviewed the causes and treatments of MCP osteoarthritis, including MCP arthritis of the thumb. A differential diagnosis of thumb MCP arthritis should include concurrent carpometacarpal osteoarthritis and sesamoid arthritis of the MCP joint.

12 Proximal Interphalangeal and Distal Interphalangeal Joint Osteoarthritis

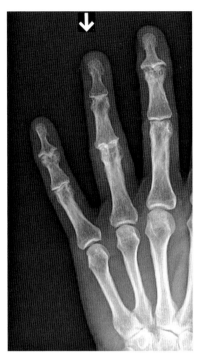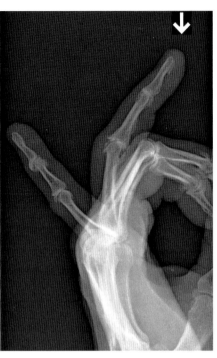

This 56-year-old woman presents to the office with a 4-year history of progressive deformity, weakness, loss of motion, pain, and tenderness localized to the proximal interphalangeal (PIP) joint of her dominant ring finger *(arrows)*. She reports no specific trauma to the finger and has been taking over-the-counter oral nonsteroidal antiinflammatory medications to control the pain. Her mother, maternal grandmother, and one sister had osteoarthritis.

Description of the Problem

Idiopathic osteoarthritis of the PIP and distal interphalangeal (DIP) joints of the fingers (and thumb) are commonly seen in older patients, but treatment is sought only rarely. The decrease in articular cartilage and the development of osteophytes and subchondral cysts occur slowly over time and are often painless. The loss of motion can affect grip strength negatively; however, this is infrequently the reason for presentation. On examination, frontal plane deformity is often present because of the asymmetrical loss of articular cartilage on the radial and ulnar surfaces of the joint and because of prominent osteophytes that prevent dorsal access to the joint for injections.

Key Anatomy

Soft tissue stabilizers of the PIP joint consist of the volar plate, the accessory collateral and proper collateral ligaments, the insertion of the central slip tendon, and the joint capsule. Stabilizers of the DIP joint are similar, but smaller in size. Although the concave shape of the base of the middle phalanx prevents dorsal translation of the middle phalanx on the head of the proximal phalanx, the joint motion is not constrained substantially by its bony anatomy.

Workup

A PA and lateral plain radiograph of the finger are all that are necessary.

Treatment

Oral nonsteroidal antiinflammatory medications are given, followed by intraarticular injections of cortico-steroids either with or without a local anesthetic. Splinting might be useful in acute flares but do not provide long-term relief for the PIP joint. Surgical treatment of the osteoarthritic PIP joint consists of either arthrodesis (using K-wires with a tension-band wire construct, a dorsal plate, or a transarticular screw) or arthroplasty (with a linked silicone prosthesis or an unlinked metal and polyethylene prosthesis). The surgical approach to the PIP joint for arthrodesis is lateral or dorsal, whereas the surgical approach to the PIP joint for arthroplasty can be volar (by detachment of the volar plate) or dorsal (by splitting of the central slip and tendon longitudinally or by a V-Y flap of the extensor tendon based distally over the insertion of the central slip). Border digits should not undergo arthroplasty, because instability results.

Surgical treatment of an osteoarthritic DIP joint consists of arthrodesis, usually using K-wires or transarticular screws. The surgical approach for DIP joint arthrodesis is through a dorsal incision for joint exposure, combined with a small incision dorsal to the nail plate for screw insertion.

Alternatives

Free transfer of a vascularized toe joint might be appropriate in rare instances of PIP arthritis. Osteotomy is rarely indicated, and excision arthroplasty leads to excessive instability in the frontal and sagittal planes. DIP splinting can be useful for treating a painful, arthritic DIP joint but will limit motion.

Principles and Clinical Pearls

- Nonoperative treatment with medication and injections is the mainstay of treatment for PIP and DIP osteoarthritis. Although intraarticular injections can be technically challenging, a 27-gauge or even a 30-gauge needle can access most joints.
- Arthrodesis of the PIP joint leads to a reliable, stable relief of pain, but it may result in concurrent DIP stiffness if the extensor mechanism develops adhesions.
- A volar approach to the PIP joint for the implantation of a PIP arthroplasty may allow earlier motion therapy postoperatively and can prevent the development of dorsal adhesions.

Pitfalls

Rheumatoid arthritis and other seropositive and seronegative arthropathies can have different natural histories and propensities for the development of deformity, bone loss, and instability. Psoriatic arthritis can cause profound digital shortening and loss of bone. Early treatment in these cases can preserve bone length.

Classic Reference

Pellegrini VD Jr, Burton RI. Osteoarthritis of the proximal interphalangeal joint of the hand: arthroplasty or fusion? J Hand Surg Am 15:194, 1990.
The authors examined patients in whom older-design arthroplasties were used. They found that arthrodesis in the radial digits and arthroplasty in the ulnar digits led to satisfactory outcomes despite bony resorption associated with silicone arthroplasties.

13 Scapholunate Advanced Collapse Wrist Arthritis

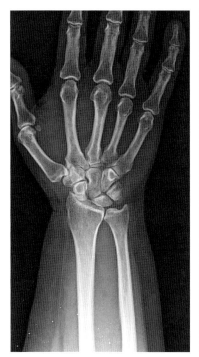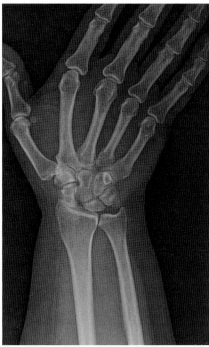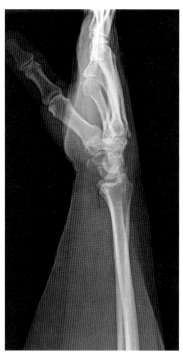

This 52-year-old executive presents to the office with a 6-year history of progressive pain, swelling, weakness, and motion loss of his right dominant wrist. He has noticed swelling over the dorsal and radial aspect of his wrist at the level of the radiocarpal joint. He recalls having been diagnosed with a wrist "sprain" while in high school, and that the associated pain and swelling lasted for approximately a month before resolving. The recent symptoms began with a minor twisting injury to the wrist sustained while taking a golfing lesson.

Description of the Problem

Disruption of the scapholunate interosseous ligament as a result of a traumatic injury (as opposed to loss of integrity from an inflammatory arthropathy such as gout, calcium pyrophosphate deposition disease, or rheumatoid arthritis) causes the scaphoid to flex and the lunate to extend. A predictable progression of styloscaphoid, radioscaphoid, and capitolunate arthritis develops, which may or may not lead to symptoms of pain, weakness, and signs of motion loss and swelling. Typically, the radiolunate joint is spared arthritic change, and the integrity of articular cartilage of this joint serves as the lynchpin for surgical reconstruction. If the proximal carpal row disruption occurs through the scaphoid, arthritis develops between the radial styloid and the scaphoid distal pole and progresses to the midcarpal joint (skipping the joint between the proximal scaphoid pole and the radius in the process).

Key Anatomy

The stability of the scaphoid is entirely from its ligamentous attachments: the dorsal scapholunate interosseous ligament, the radioscaphocapitate ligament volarly, and the ligamentous attachment to the trapezium and trapezoid distally. If these stabilizers are disrupted, the scaphoid will undergo obligate flexion, and the contact pressure between the scaphoid and the radius and radial styloid will increase. The radioscaphoid angle will increase and lead to cartilage loss and the development of joint space narrowing, subchondral sclerosis, and radial styloid osteophytes. Arthritis, occasionally symptomatic, results.

Workup

Once arthritis develops between the scaphoid and the radius, only plain PA and lateral radiographs are needed. MRI or arthrographic imaging can be useful (as can arthroscopic evaluation) if a surgical reconstruction is planned to preserve the joint between the scaphoid fossa of the distal radius and the proximal pole of the scaphoid.

Treatment

Nonoperative treatment with oral antiinflammatory drugs, splinting, and activity modification are attempted initially. If these do not successfully alleviate pain and increase grip strength, surgical treatment is considered. If the radioscaphoid joint appears nonarthritic, then scaphotrapeziotrapezoid arthrodesis with a radial styloidectomy can be performed. If the radioscaphoid joint is arthritic, then either excision or arthrodesis of this joint is performed. Total wrist fusion, total wrist arthroplasty, scaphoid excision with a four-corner fusion, and proximal row carpectomy are options. If a chronic scaphoid nonunion has led to the development of radioscaphoid arthritis in the absence of capitolunate arthritis, excision of the distal pole of the scaphoid along with radial styloidectomy is considered.

Alternatives

Proximal-row carpectomy has been combined with an interposition arthroplasty of the dorsal capsule in cases in which a proximal-row carpectomy is planned and the head of the capitate is arthritic. In some patients who do not wish to have complex surgery, wrist denervation may limit the pain.

Principles and Clinical Pearls

- If the scaphoid is fixed in flexion on initial presentation, then preservation of the radioscaphoid joint by surgical repositioning of the scaphoid (either by capsulodesis or arthrodesis) will fail.
- Any treatment of capitolunate arthritis that does not include excision or arthrodesis of this joint will have a poor result.
- Patients often present after a minor mishap that occurred decades after the initial injury. Their symptoms typically resolve after a period of immobilization and medication. Reconstructive surgery for these patients is not recommended.

Pitfalls

Failure to address an arthritic joint by excision arthroplasty, implant arthroplasty, or arthrodesis will lead to inconsistent and unpredictable results after surgical treatment.

Classic Reference

Watson HK, Ballet FL. The SLAC wrist: scapholunate advanced collapse pattern of degenerative arthritis. J Hand Surg Am 9:358, 1984.
This was the initial manuscript that described the development of the pattern of SLAC wrist arthritis, by the surgeon who is credited with describing the scaphoid shift test.

14 Metacarpophalangeal Joint Rheumatoid Arthritis

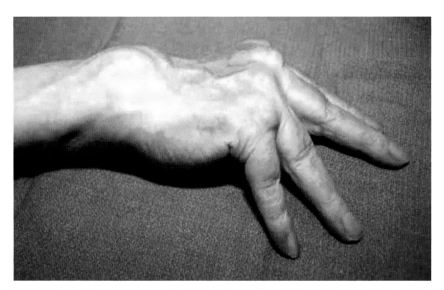

This 57-year-old woman presents to the office with a history of rheumatoid arthritis, diagnosed 20 years previously. She has been treated with oral corticosteroids and disease-modifying antirheumatic drugs, both with limited success. Over the past 3 years she has noticed a progressive deformity of her metacarpophalangeal (MCP) joints of both hands that causes the fingers to be deviated ulnarly at the MCP joints and the thumb MCP joint to be floppy and unable to grip or pinch. The deformity is aesthetically displeasing to her; however, the pain and the dysfunction associated with the arthritis of these joints are the primary reasons for her seeking surgical attention. Although her thumb is unstable, it is not painful. (Photo courtesy of James W. Strickland, MD.)

Description of the Problem

Ulnar deviation at the MCP joints can lead to weakness of grip and pinch, pain, tenderness, loss of function and dexterity, and aesthetic compromise. Surgical treatment involves a rebalancing of forces across the MCP joint and includes recentralization of the long extensor tendons, plication of the radial sagittal band and the radial collateral ligaments at the MCP level, transection or recession of the ulnar intrinsics (including the abductor digiti minimi hypothenar muscle-tendon unit), and synovectomy of the joint. Surgeons disagree on whether concurrent radiocarpal procedures should be performed in the absence of symptoms localized to that joint.

Key Anatomy

The exact pathogenesis of the development of the ulnar drift deformity seen commonly in the hands of rheumatoid patients is not known. At present, it is thought that the development of radiocarpal synovitis and the subsequent weakening of the extrinsic volar wrist ligaments lead to ulnar translocation of the carpus and an obligate radial deviation of the metacarpus. The intact long flexor and extensor tendons maintain their longitudinal direction of pull toward the base of fibrous flexor sheath and the base of the middle phalanx, respectively, thereby exerting an ulnar-directed pull on the MCP joints, whose collateral ligament support and volar plates are weakened by articular synovitis. If the process progresses, the volar support of the MCP joints is lost, and the base of the proximal phalanx subluxes volar to the head of the metacarpal. The extensor tendons, if intact, become permanently located ulnar to the metacarpal head, and active MCP extension is lost.

Workup

The cervical spine, shoulders, and elbows are evaluated. The peripheral nerves are examined (especially the posterior interosseous nerve), and the continuity of the extensor tendons is assessed (especially the long extensors to the fourth and fifth fingers) in case tendon transfer is needed to treat a caput ulnae syndrome. An unstable cervical spine will affect anesthesia, and stiff or unstable shoulder or elbow joints will affect positioning intraoperatively. PA and lateral plain radiographs of the hand and wrist are evaluated for the previously described pathology. In particular, the degree of bony destruction from periarticular synovitis is noted. If a patient takes medications for rheumatoid arthritis that affect the immune system adversely or soft tissue healing, then consultation preoperatively with the prescribing rheumatologist is needed.

Treatment

Nonsurgical treatment will not arrest or modify the disease process; it will only delay the surgical correction if the patient is disabled. Surgery involves MCP joint replacement using linked silicone prostheses and soft tissue rebalancing about the MCP joint, as described previously. Wrist stabilization procedures are performed concurrently if indicated. Either a total wrist fusion or a radiolunate fusion (a Chamay fusion) is performed to stabilize the carpus and metacarpus, to arrest progression of ulnar carpal translocation, and to allow definitive MCP soft tissue rebalancing to occur. Thumb MCP instability is treated surgically by fusion either with a K-wire and tension-band wire construct or a dorsal plate and screws.

Alternatives

In rare instances, soft tissue rebalancing and limited wrist arthrodesis (a Chamay radiolunate fusion) can be performed in early stages of the disease to arrest its progression. Tendon transfers of the long wrist extensors are carried out to recentralize the lunate in the lunate fossa of the distal radius and to arrest ulnar deviation have not gained favor.

Principles and Clinical Pearls

- Postoperative dynamic extension splinting with the slings placed in slight radial deviation allows a stable and mobile soft tissue envelope to develop around the arthroplasties.
- The prostheses themselves should be thought of as interpositions, rather than implant arthroplasties. They maintain the position of the finger with respect to the metacarpal and effect proper soft tissue tension to promote active digital flexion and passive digital extension at the MCP joints.

Pitfalls

The use of too-small arthroplasties can lead to MCP joint subluxation or dislocation. The use of unlinked prostheses can cause similar complications.

Classic Reference

Goldfarb CA, Stern PJ. Metacarpophalangeal joint arthroplasty in rheumatoid arthritis. A long-term assessment. J Bone Joint Surg Am 85:1869, 2013.
Two hundred and eight arthroplasties in 52 hands of 36 patients were evaluated, and the long-term results were found to deteriorate with time. Almost two thirds of implants were broken, and only a quarter of hands were pain free. The authors suggested that further advancement in the treatment of this manifestation of rheumatoid arthritis was going to be medical rather than surgical.

15 Pisotriquetral Joint Osteoarthritis

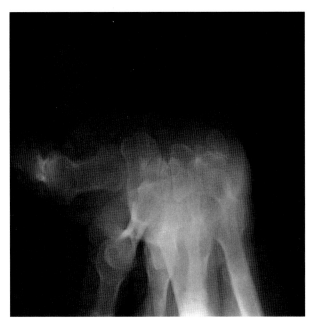

This is a carpal tunnel view of a 64-year-old real estate agent who has a 6-month history of progressive ulnar-sided wrist and hand pain and tenderness. She has increased pain and tenderness when she does yoga, especially in positions in which she places weight on the proximal aspect of the palm of her hand. She has no history of trauma. On examination, she has tenderness on palpation of her pisotriquetral joint and on palpation of her pisiform. Ulnar nerve–innervated muscles in her hand are at full strength, and blood flow through the ulnar artery is normal (volar arterial flow is through two intact arches). Radiograph demonstrates a narrow pisotriquetral joint with subchondral sclerosis taken as an obliquely positioned radiograph.

Description of the Problem

Loss of articular cartilage between the dorsal aspect of the pisiform and the volar aspect of the triquetrum can become symptomatic. Pisotriquetral osteoarthritis is a relatively uncommon cause for ulnar-sided wrist and hand pain. It can usually be diagnosed by plain radiographs. A differential diagnosis includes a pisiform or hook of hamate fracture (see Chapter 53), a lunotriquetral ligament tear, triangular fibrocartilage complex degeneration or tear, extensor carpi ulnaris tendonitis or subluxation, midcarpal instability, an ulnar canal ganglion, or an ulnar artery thrombosis or ganglion. A diagnosis is based on clinical examination and plain radiographic confirmation using either a carpal tunnel view (see figure) or a semisupinated lateral view of the wrist.

Key Anatomy

The ulnar nerve and ulnar artery pass radial to the pisiform as they enter the Guyon canal. Contained within the tendinous insertion of the flexor carpi radialis, the pisiform functions as a sesamoid bone to increase the mechanical advantage of wrist flexion and ulnar deviation. The articular surface of the pisotriquetral joint is broad, and access for injection of a corticosteroid is aided by fluoroscopic localization of the joint and access from the ulnar side. The dorsal cutaneous branch of the ulnar nerve is most frequently dorsal over the body of the triquetrum at the level of the pisotriquetral joint and is not in danger of injection or laceration during exposure.

Workup

PA, lateral, and either a carpal tunnel view of the wrist or a semisupinated lateral view of the wrist are most useful.

Treatment

Activity modification, a forearm-based splint (either custom-molded or off-the-shelf), oral antiinflammatory agents given on a scheduled basis, and/or fluoroscopy-assisted intraarticular injections of a corticosteroid with or without a local anesthetic are the initial treatments. Injections can be repeated as necessary. The injection of hyaluronate has not proved significantly beneficial. Operative treatment can be performed in patients whose symptoms are unrelieved by nonoperative means. Pisiform excision is performed in these patients.

Alternatives

There are no surgical treatments other than pisiform excision.

Principles and Clinical Pearls

- Diagnosing ulnar-sided wrist pain can be challenging. The distinguishing feature of these patients is tenderness over the pisiform, combined with radiographic signs of cartilage loss and arthritis.
- Intraoperative dissection of the ulnar nerve and ulnar artery through the Guyon canal is essential to prevent injury to these longitudinally running structures. The deep motor branch of the ulnar nerve exits the nerve on its ulnar aspect and then curves deep to the nerve while traveling in an ulnar direction.

Pitfalls

Complications of surgical excision of the pisiform include injury to the ulnar nerve or the ulnar artery.

Classic Reference

Johnson GH, Tonkin MA. Excision of pisiform in pisotriquetral arthritis. Clin Orthop Relat Res 210:137, 1986.
In seven of eight patients treated, excision of the pisiform combined with release of the Guyon canal and ulnar nerve isolation and decompression led to relief of symptoms.

16 Posttraumatic Wrist Arthritis

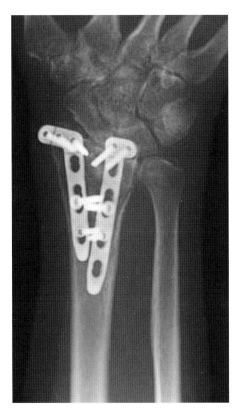

This 43-year-old manual laborer has a mutifragmentary intraarticular distal radius fracture caused by a work-related injury 3 years previously. He had an uncomplicated course after reduction, fixation, immobilization, and rehabilitation and returned to heavy labor 4 months after the initial injury. Over the past 9 months, he has had increasing pain, swelling, loss of motion, and loss of strength related to his wrist. On examination, he has tenderness on palpation of the radiocarpal joint dorsally and volarly. His wrist range of motion is limited and painful in all planes. His grip strength testing shows decreased strength at all positions of the device, and pinch strength is decreased on the contralateral side.

Description of the Problem

Posttraumatic arthritis of the radiocarpal joint is common after an intraarticular fracture of the distal radius. Although several authors have posited that reduction of the articular surface to a step or gap deformity of less than 2 mm can prevent the development of osteoarthritis, whether posttraumatic arthritis is painful or affects function negatively is debatable. Articular incongruity in the scaphoid fossa, the lunate fossa, or the sigmoid notch can increase cartilage contact pressures and lead to cartilage degradation, but most patients are functionally well and require little active treatment. The mainstays of treatment are oral nonsteroidal antiinflammatory drugs and intermittent splint immobilization and corticosteroid injections. These can decrease symptoms satisfactorily to allow surgical treatment to be deferred.

Key Anatomy

The proximal pole and waist of the scaphoid articulate with the radial styloid and the scaphoid fossa of the distal radius. The proximal pole of the lunate articulates with the lunate fossa of the distal radius and the seat of the ulna. Any or all of these joints can become arthritic, and symptoms vary depending on whether the wrist or the forearm is involved primarily.

Workup

Plain radiographs should be evaluated, including PA, lateral, ulnar deviation, and supinated clenched fist views of the wrist. A CT scan to evaluate the presence or absence of arthritic change in the three potential articular locations can be obtained for preoperative planning if an intraarticular osteotomy is considered. In general, CT scans and MRI are not helpful. An injection of a local anesthetic under fluoroscopic guidance might be useful to determine the primary location of the pain. A trial of casting or other form of immobilization can help to determine how well a patient will tolerate arthrodesis. Electrophysiologic testing should be carried out if a total wrist arthrodesis is considered, given the recommendation by some authors that concurrent carpal tunnel release (CTR) be done at the time of arthrodesis to prevent the development of a postoperative acute carpal tunnel syndrome that would require emergent decompression.

Treatment

Initial treatment includes activity modification, a forearm-based splint (either custom-molded or off-the-shelf), and oral antiinflammatory agents given on a scheduled basis. Corticosteroid injections can be given for short-term pain control. Operative treatment is reserved for patients whose symptoms are unrelieved by nonoperative means. In these patients, a total wrist arthrodesis provides pain relief and a reliable return to functional activity. If some motion is desirable, then a radioscapholunate arthrodesis can be performed with or without an excision of the distal pole of the scaphoid to unlock the midcarpal joint. A total wrist arthroplasty is another option, but its long-term durability is questionable in younger patients and in those involved in lifting heavy weights.

Alternatives

Interposition arthroplasty of the dorsal capsule has been attempted, and interposition of a fascia lata autograft or allograft has been performed for radiocarpal and distal radioulnar joint arthritis.

Principles and Clinical Pearls

- Total wrist arthrodesis should be paired with a low threshold for considering CTR or distal radioulnar joint resection. Postoperative immobilization of the wrist will prevent any appreciable flexor tendon bow-stringing and should resolve many local aggravations that occur after CTR such as scar tenderness and pillar pain.
- Most patients with posttraumatic arthritis of the wrist do well without surgical treatment and show normal or near-normal scores on the Disabilities of the Arm, Shoulder, and Hand Outcome Measure.

Pitfalls

Radioscapholunate fusion is technically difficult and should be performed only in patients in whom motion is not only desirable but also required.

Classic Reference

Hastings H II, Weiss AP, Quenzer D, Wiedeman GP, Hanington KR, Strickland JW. Arthrodesis of the wrist for post-traumatic disorders. J Bone Joint Surg Am 78:897, 1996.
In a series of ninety sequential total wrist fusions, the authors described improved reliability and shorter time to successful fusion in patients treated with plate fixation, compared with other methods of fixation.

17 Ulnar Impaction Syndrome

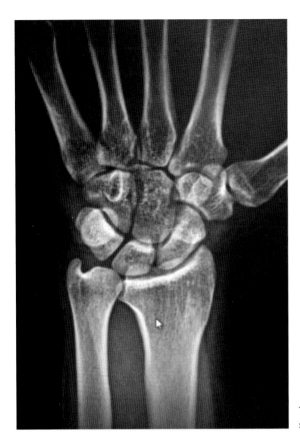

This patient had right ulnar-sided wrist pain. A PA radiograph shows a long ulna compared with the radius.

Description of the Problem

The radiograph shows that the patient has ulnar positive variance. Evidence indicates that the patient may have had a distal radius fracture in the past, which has affected the growth and led to ulnar positive variance and compression of the triangular fibrocartilage complex (TFCC).

Key Anatomy

The radius and ulna at the level of the proximal row should have equal length, distributing load across both bones. In this case, the patient has 3 to 4 mm of ulnar positive variance. The increased length of the ulna begins to cause impingement of the TFCC with the lunate. Over time, the TFCC can be injured, with changes to the cartilage of the lunate. This results in ulnar-sided wrist pain.

Workup

The patient should be evaluated for ulnar-sided wrist pain, ruling out other causes, including pisotriquetral arthritis (see Chapter 15), lunotriquetral ligament tear, extensor carpi ulnaris and flexor carpi ulnaris tendonitis, and subluxation of the extensor carpi ulnaris tendon. Surgeons can compare the length of the radius and ulna on radiographs. An MRI is performed to assess the TFCC and the lunate. Palpation on the volar side of the ulnar wrist helps to evaluate tenderness over the TFCC. The position of the distal ulna should be assessed. Subluxation of the distal radioulnar joint and pain are determined by shucking the distal radioulnar joint. This highlights distal radioulnar joint arthritis and global instability.

Treatment

The standard treatment for ulnar impaction syndrome is wrist arthroscopy to assess and possibly debride the TFCC, followed by an ulnar-shortening osteotomy. Shortening is performed through a longitudinal incision over the midportion of the ulna, using one of the various ulnar-shortening sets. This decreases the load across the proximal row. The shape of the distal radioulnar joint is examined to ensure the shortening does not cause distal radioulnar joint incongruity. An ulnar-shortening osteotomy needs to be technically precise to decrease the chance of a nonunion. This procedure should not be undertaken in smokers because of the increased risk of nonunion of this thick cortical bone.

Alternatives

This procedure has many alternatives. Some patients who do not want the attendant risks of and long-term immobilization required for an ulnar-shortening osteotomy may elect to undergo wrist arthroscopy and TFCC debridement only. These patients should be informed that a shortening osteotomy may be required if symptoms persist. A corrective osteotomy of the radius may be necessary in patients with a severe fracture and malunion of the distal radius. Several salvage operations are available, including an arthroscopic wafer, whereby the distal ulna is debrided through an arthroscopic approach; an open hemiresection of the distal ulna; a Darrach procedure in which the distal ulna is excised; and a Sauve-Kapandji procedure in which the distal radioulnar joint is fused and the proximal ulna is released to allow pronation and supination. All of these salvage procedures have risks of destabilizing the normal anatomy.

Principles and Clinical Pearls

- Radiographs are critical to assess the length of the ulna versus the length of the radius in patients with ulnar-sided wrist pain.
- Although an ulnar-shortening osteotomy is the preferred procedure, many patients do not want the risks and lengthy immobilization that is necessary.
- Salvage operations such as those listed previously may be effective in relieving pain but have the added risk of contorting normal anatomy and destabilizing the wrist.

Pitfalls

Pitfalls include persistent pain, nonunion of the ulna, incongruity of the distal radioulnar joint, and progressive wrist destabilization. Specifically, the ulnar-shortening osteotomy technique needs to be precise. A nonunion is a very difficult problem to address because of the minimal amount of cancellous bone in the area.

Classic References

McBeath R, Katolik LI, Shin EK. Ulnar shortening osteotomy for ulnar impaction syndrome. J Hand Surg Am 38:379, 2013.
Dr. McBeath and her colleagues presented a short, evidence-based review of ulnar-shortening osteotomy, including the workup for ulnar-sided wrist pain.

Stockton DJ, Pelletier ME, Pike JM. Operative treatment of ulnar impaction syndrome: a systematic review. J Hand Surg Eur Vol 40:470, 2015.
This was an interesting systematic review of operative treatment of ulnar impaction syndrome that described multiple procedures. The authors concluded that an arthroscopic wafer procedure and an open hemiresection procedure may be viable alternatives to an ulnar-shortening osteotomy.

Burns

18 Thermal Burn

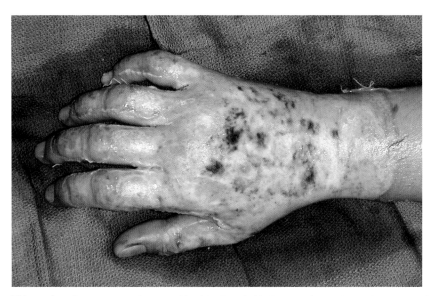

This patient has a severe burn to his right hand. He is seen in the intensive care unit 2 hours after the injury.

Description of the Problem

The patient has a severe burn of either deep partial thickness or full thickness to the right hand. He needs immediate management consisting of escharatomy, possible fasciotomy, and dressing changes, with anticipation of early debridement and grafting.

Key Anatomy

In patients with deep partial-thickness or full-thickness burns, the level of depth may be hard to determine at the time of injury. However, if circumferential burns are present around the finger and hand, the patient will need emergent escharatomy to release the tightened scar and allow blood flow to the fingers. If the swelling becomes severe, hand compartment release may be necessary. Deep partial-thickness and full-thickness burns are relatively insensate. The depth of a burn injury will determine the need for grafting versus flap coverage.

Workup

Patients with deep burns to the hand require care in a designated burn unit. A workup will include obtaining the history of the injury. Patients with injuries that occurred in a closed-space environment may also have inhalational injury. Burns isolated to the hand require immediate focus on the need for an escharatomy or fasciotomy. Pain control and fluid resuscitation are critical. Dressing changes are begun with silver sulfadiazine (Silvadene), which will penetrate the eschar. Splinting is critical initially.

Treatment

A splint is placed with the hand in a position of safety and the wrist extended 30 degrees, the metacarpophalangeal joints flexed 90 degrees, and the interphalangeal joints straight. Escharatomies are performed in the fingers along the noncontact sides. If necessary, escharatomies are performed along the midlateral lines bilaterally to each digit. Early tangential excision and skin grafting are important. With a tourniquet in place, the skin is tangentially excised until healthy punctate bleeding occurs. If the need for grafting is questionable, dressings or allograft or xenograft skin may be used as a temporary cover. Definitive grafting should be performed with split-thickness skin grafting if the area is extensive and with full-thickness grafting if it is small. Often, an unmeshed skin graft can be placed, which would lead to comparable take rates and a better aesthetic result.

Alternatives

There are no alternatives to tangential excision and grafting. If a wound is full thickness and involves deeper structures, including the extensor tendons, then flaps may be necessary.

Principles and Clinical Pearls

- Immediate management consists of stabilization of the patient, escharatomies, and fasciotomies as needed.
- Splinting is critical to prevent burn contracture initially and postoperatively.
- Tangential excision is performed until good punctate bleeding is noted, then skin grafting is performed.

Pitfalls

There are many pitfalls with complex burn injuries to the hand. An understanding of the need for resuscitation in a designated burn unit is essential. If escharatomies are not performed, then digits may be threatened. Many burn injuries lead to significant contractures if attention is not paid to excision, grafting, and postoperative splinting with therapy.

Classic References

Fufa D, Chuang SS, Yang JY. Postburn contractures of the hand. J Hand Surg Am 39:1869, 2014.
If hand burns are not properly treated, postburn contractures can result. This review article classified the various burn injuries that may develop, with algorithms for treatment.

Prasetyono TO, Sadikin PM, Saputra DK. The use of split-thickness versus full-thickness skin graft to resurface volar aspect of pediatric burned hands: a systematic review. Burns 41:890, 2015.
In many cases, full-thickness skin grafting has been favored as opposed to split-thickness skin grafting for resurfacing the volar aspect of the hands. In this systematic review, the authors found that both graft types were useful, and that no data showed full-thickness skin grafting to be superior for covering pediatric volar burns.

19 Delayed Burn Reconstruction

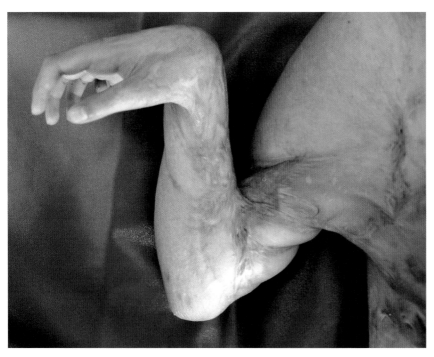

This teenage girl had a severe flame burn that occurred several years ago. She is seen in an overseas outreach clinic with this burn contracture. She has had one previous skin grafting procedure.

Description of the Problem

The patient has a severe burn contracture involving her entire right upper extremity. She has tightness in her axilla, elbow, wrist, and hand. This will require extensive scar release and either a skin graft or flap reconstruction.

Key Anatomy

Severe flame burns cause deep partial-thickness or full-thickness burns. The subcutaneous tissue can also be involved if the burns are severe. Over time, as the skin contracts to heal the wound, the joints may be deformed as the power of scar contracture becomes evident. This upper extremity posture severely limits the use of the hand.

Workup

Each joint in this patient's extremity must be evaluated for active and passive range of motion. Palpation of the skin will reveal where the scar is most tight and requires release. A good understanding of how the problem evolved is critical to the outcome of the procedure. Were skin grafts performed early? Were physical therapy and splinting adequate after surgery? Does the patient have other burn areas that will limit skin grafting and flap reconstruction? Do the patient and family understand the dedication to splinting and hand therapy that is required after surgery? Is the patient's nutritional and emotional status appropriate for surgical intervention?

Treatment

The operation will require a significant scar release with skin grafting and/or flap reconstruction. Because multiple joints are involved, one or two joints are chosen for release in an initial procedure, and a plan is developed for progressive releases. Each joint that is released may require additional surgery. Scarring and fusion of the joints over time should be anticipated. Therefore radiographs are critical to evaluate each joint. In this case, the patient noted that the elbow flexion was the greatest cause of disability. Thus the elbow was planned for initial release. The tight scar band is carefully palpated and released. The underlying brachial artery, median nerve, and ulnar nerve are carefully identified and protected. Once the scar bands are released, a large soft tissue area will need coverage. This should be anticipated. A split-thickness skin graft is the first line of treatment in this complex operation. However, surgeons must be prepared for regional or free flaps in case the dissection results in exposed nerves and blood vessels. Split-thickness skin grafts can be harvested from the thighs or other areas of unburned skin. For flap reconstruction, a fasciocutaneous flap or a muscle flap can be used, and the vessel anastomosed end to side to the brachial artery. Veins must be carefully found, because they may have been involved in the initial burn. Blood loss should be minimized with the use of a tourniquet, epinephrine, and careful, meticulous hemostasis. Once the joint is released and covered, an elbow extension splint is placed.

Alternatives

The major alternative is the decision to proceed with surgery at this time. If the patient is not adequately supported with physical therapy after surgery, then surgery can be futile because the wound will recontract in this way. The patient should be carefully counseled that multiple-stage procedures may be necessary. The scar release itself is standard; however, alternatives for skin coverage are numerous, ranging from split-thickness skin grafts to full-thickness skin grafts to regional and free flaps.

Principles and Clinical Pearls

- Adequate physical therapy and emotional support are necessary before beginning delayed burn reconstruction.
- The surgeon should ask the patient which joint would create better function. Based on this response, multiple operative stages should be planned.
- After skin is released, the underlying structures need to be carefully identified and preserved.
- The amount of skin coverage needed after scar release should not be underestimated.

Pitfalls

Major pitfalls are associated with this complex operation. Joint release may be difficult because of severe involvement of the tendons and capsular tissue underlying the scar contracture. Major nerves and arteries are in harm's way because of the depth of the burn. The amount of skin coverage needed is frequently underestimated. Therefore, because of the amount of skin coverage and blood loss and the length of the operation, one joint should be released at each operation.

Classic References

Cartotto R, Cicuto BJ, Kiwanuka HN, Bueno EM, Pomahac B. Common postburn deformities and their management. Surg Clin North Am 94:817, 2014.
This was a review article of postburn deformities and management. Because of the nature of burn reconstruction, with each operation being unique, very few large clinical trials have been conducted. This paper presented axillary release, elbow release, and hand release, with excellent photographs.

McKee DM. Reconstructive options of burn injuries to the hand and upper extremity. J Hand Surg Am 36:922, 2011.
This excellent review of reconstructive options for burn injuries to the hand and upper extremity discussed immediate escharotomy, fasciotomy, and a variety of subacute and late reconstructive options.

Omar MT, Hassan AA. Evaluation of hand function after early excision and skin grafting of burns versus delayed skin grafting: a randomized clinical trial. Burns 37:707, 2011.
This study from Egypt compared early excision and grafting versus delayed burn skin grafting for hand function. They logically concluded that early excision and skin grafting with physiotherapy led to better results.

Compartment Syndromes

20 Compartment Syndrome

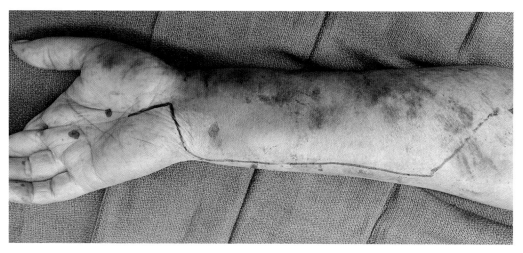

This 20-year-old male student fell onto his outstretched right arm while skateboarding. He had acute fractures of the midshaft of the radius and the ulna. A splint was placed in the emergency department. The patient was taken to the operating room the following day for open reduction and internal fixation of the fractures. He was given a general anesthetic for the procedure. That evening he had pain in his forearm and was unable to flex or extend his fingers and thumb actively. His peripheral pulses were present and palpable; however, sensation was subjectively altered over the entire volar and dorsal aspects of his hand and wrist. On palpation of his volar and dorsal forearm, the muscles were tense, hard, and noncompressible, and direct pressure on the forearm was extremely painful. A pressure monitor showed elevated volar and dorsal intramuscular pressures. The patient was taken to the operating room.

Description of the Problem

Posttraumatic compartment syndrome is a surgical emergency. The three *P*s of diagnosis are pain (at rest and especially on passive stretch of the affected compartment), pressure (increased on palpation and subjectively), and paresthesias (from peripheral sensory nerve ischemia). Pallor, pulselessness, and paralysis occur infrequently and are not reliable for confirming or ruling out the diagnosis.

Key Anatomy

A *compartment* is defined as an osteofascial space of fixed volume. The forearm has a superficial compartment containing the pronator teres, flexor carpi radialis, palmaris longus, and flexor carpi ulnaris muscles and several deep compartments containing the flexor digitorum superficialis, the flexor digitorum profundus and flexor pollicis longus, and the peroneus quartus muscle. (The exact number of deep compartments is two or three, depending on whether the fascial boundary between the flexor digitorum superficialis and flexor digitorum profundus/flexor pollicis longus muscle belly is considered.). An additional compartment containing the mobile wad of the brachioradialis, the extensor carpi radialis longus, and the extensor carpi radialis brevis muscles is located dorsally, along with one other dorsal compartment containing the extensor digitorum communis muscle bellies and the outcropper muscles (abductor pollicis longus and extensor pollicis brevis). The brachial artery and median nerve are immediately subjacent to the bicipital biceps aponeurosis proximally and are at risk of iatrogenic injury during proximal compartment release. The location of the median nerve in the superficial radial aspect of the carpal tunnel and of the ulnar nerve in the deep ulnar aspect of Guyon's canal is noted during decompression. The location of the palmar cutaneous branch of the median nerve, between the flexor carpi radialis and the palmaris longus tendons at the level of the wrist, is noted to prevent iatrogenic injury.

Workup

If pressure within the compartment is elevated for any reason such as trauma, hematoma (from anticoagulation or trauma), an abscess, or infiltration of administered fluids, then surgical decompression must be performed emergently. Although opinions differ on what constitutes elevated pressure, the presence of an intracompartmental pressure higher than 30 mm Hg or the presence of classical signs and symptoms should steer surgeons toward compartment release. Clinical suspicion and erring on the side of release rather than observation are recommended in questionable clinical presentations, such as those with concurrent nerve injury or anesthetic blocks, and in patients unable to communicate the presence of pain, pressure, or paresthesias, such as those with closed head injuries.

Treatment

Surgical release of the compartments affected is the only treatment. Proximally the bicipital biceps aponeurosis is released, thus relieving pressure on the median nerve and brachial artery, and distally the carpal tunnel is released. The incision is started distally as for a standard carpal tunnel release and is carried ulnarly at the level of the wrist crease. The incision is continued proximally along the volar ulnar aspect of the forearm and across the elbow in a zigzag fashion. Primary wound closure is rarely recommended except over the carpal tunnel as a protection for the exposed median nerve. Split-thickness skin grafts meshed 1:1.5 are used for wound coverage, along with a negative-pressure dressing if appropriate.

Alternatives

In rare instances in which the intracompartmental pressure is within the normal range, the patient may be carefully observed for a period of time in the hope of resolution. If in doubt, surgeons should perform an urgent or emergent fasciotomy.

Principles and Clinical Pearls

- A forearm fasciotomy should include a carpal tunnel release, a brachial artery and proximal median nerve release, superficial and deep volar compartment release, and a mobile wad release through a dorsal incision if indicated.
- Split-thickness skin grafting after compartment release should be done as soon as it is practical.

Pitfalls

A missed diagnosis because of inattention or confounding signs or symptoms can lead to a Volkmann's ischemic contracture. This is a clinical disaster that requires reconstructive surgery that can include muscle debridements and contracture releases, nerve decompressions, tendon transfers, and potentially even free-functioning muscle transfer to restore active digital flexion. In this condition more than any other (with the possible exception of an acute carpal tunnel syndrome), early diagnosis and treatment is critical for a successful clinical outcome.

Classic Reference

Friedrich JB, Shin AY. Management of forearm compartment syndrome. Hand Clin 23:245, 2007.
This review article discussed diagnosis and treatment of forearm compartment syndrome, a surgically emergent complication of injury and treatment.

21 Acute Carpal Tunnel Syndrome

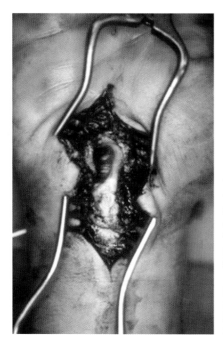

This 24-year-old man presented to the emergency department after a fall from the top of an 8-foot ladder while at work. He landed on his outstretched right arm and hyperextended his right wrist. He had pain immediately in his wrist and began to note increased pain in his hand and altered sensation in the thumb, index, middle, and ring finger within a short period of time. A half hour later, an examination reveals a dense anesthesia in the median nerve distribution and paralysis of his thenar muscles. He has profound swelling volarly and dorsally and a positive Tinel sign on percussion of the median nerve in the distal forearm and at the carpal tunnel. Plain radiographs demonstrate a dorsal perilunate dislocation with the lunate tipped volarly out of the lunate fossa and the capitate resting in the lunate fossa of the distal radius.

Description of the Problem

High-energy trauma to the hand, carpus, or distal forearm can lead to an emergent elevation in pressure within the carpal tunnel. Resting carpal tunnel pressure is 4 mm Hg or less; however, in acute carpal tunnel syndrome, the pressure can exceed 100 mm Hg and cause extreme pain and lead to paresthesia, anesthesia, and paralysis of median nerve–innervated musculature. The emergent treatment involves reduction and realignment of any displaced fracture or dislocation and decompression of the median nerve at the carpal tunnel if signs and symptoms of median nerve compression do not resolve immediately.

Key Anatomy

The carpal tunnel is bordered by the carpal arch and the transverse carpal ligament. Division of the transverse carpal ligament causes a 24% increase in the volume of the carpal tunnel by means of anterior displacement of the median nerve and the tendons contained therein and does not widen the bony carpal arch.

Workup

PA, lateral, ulnar deviation, and supinated clenched fist plain radiographs of the wrist are reviewed. If compartment syndrome of the forearm or the hand is suspected, appropriate pressure readings are obtained in the forearm compartments and the interosseous, thenar, and hypothenar compartments (see Chapter 20).

Treatment

Emergent closed reduction of any fracture or dislocation should be performed to realign the wrist and increase carpal tunnel volume. If symptom relief is incomplete after reduction, emergent operative carpal tunnel release must be undertaken. Operative fixation of bony and ligamentous injuries can be performed at the same operative setting. However, it should not take precedence over release of the transverse carpal ligament through an incision of sufficient length to visualize the entire median nerve through the traumatized field, which may alter the nerve's expected position with respect to the usual landmarks.

Alternatives

There are no alternative treatments.

Principles and Clinical Pearls

- Acute carpal tunnel syndrome is a surgical emergency: All deformities are reduced immediately. If symptoms do not resolve, then operative extensile carpal tunnel release with or without bony fixation of associated fractures or dislocations should be undertaken.
- Compartment release of the forearm or the hand should be performed at the same surgical setting. The tourniquet is inflated for only a short time to aid in visualization of the important neural structures, but after decompression, the tourniquet is deflated to allow perfusion of the previously ischemic nerve.

Pitfalls

Complications of surgery include delayed recovery and iatrogenic injury to the palmar cutaneous branch of the median nerve, the recurrent motor branch of the median nerve, and the superficial carpal arch. Of these structures, only the superficial arch should be visualized routinely during emergent carpal tunnel release.

Classic Reference

Szabo RM. Acute carpal tunnel syndrome. Hand Clin 14:419, 1998.
A variety of traumatic, hematologic, and infectious conditions can cause acute carpal tunnel syndrome. The treatment is release of the transverse carpal ligament.

Congenital Conditions

22 Thumb Polydactyly

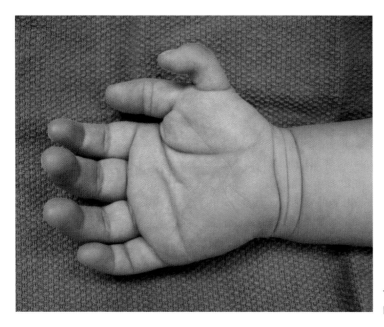

This patient has right type IV thumb polydactyly.

Description of the Problem

The patient has polydactyly. Most families wish for surgical excision. Treatment requires more of a reconstruction than a simple excision.

Key Anatomy

The classic categorization of polydactyly is the Wassel classification. In this progressive classification, type I is a bifid distal phalanx. Type II is two separate distal phalanges, type III is a bifid proximal phalanx and two separate distal phalanges, type IV is two separate proximal phalanges and two separate distal phalanges, type V is type IV with a bifid metacarpal, and type VI is two separate metacarpals and separate phalanges distally. Type IV is most common.

Workup

As with any congenital anomaly, syndromes or associated anomalies are ruled out. Thumb polydactyly is usually an isolated anomaly. Radiographs are obtained just before surgery. It is unnecessary to obtain radiographs early, because they are not useful until the time of surgery, usually when the child is 10 to 12 months of age.

Treatment

Type IV polydactyly has a bifid proximal phalanx and distal phalanx but a common metacarpal bone. The radial thumb is usually smaller and will be sacrificed, because the ulnar collateral ligament to the thumb is critical. This procedure is not merely removal of the extra thumb. Both the thumb to be removed and the thumb to be retained are anatomically dissected, because the flexor and extensor tendons may cause deviation of the digit and require release and/or transfer. The operation begins with an incision along the proximal phalanx of the radial thumb to be removed. Extra skin is preserved initially to prevent a shortage of skin. The incision is designed laterally over the thenar space and distally into the normal ulnar thumb. The extensor and flexor tendon to the radial thumb are dissected and followed as they proceed ulnarly. The abductor pollicis brevis muscle usually inserts onto the radial thumb, and this should be dissected off and tagged. The radial collateral ligament to the extra thumb is dissected free and tagged. The surgeon decides whether to centralize the flexor and extensor tendons, with possible tendon transfer from the digit to be removed. The radial-sided thumb is removed. The metacarpal head should be broader and is reduced with an osteotome to minimize bulk. The radial collateral ligament at the proximal metacarpal head is then attached to the ulnar-sided thumb, and the abductor pollicis brevis muscle is resuspended onto the ulnar-sided thumb. Skin flaps are rearranged in a zigzag fashion, and the skin is closed.

Alternatives

In cases in which the thumbs are the same size, the decision of which one to remove is critical. This should be carefully communicated to the family. However, in most cases, the ulnar-sided thumb is retained, and the radial-sided thumb is removed. In some situations, because of cultural reasons or family preference, no polydactyly excision is performed.

Principles and Clinical Pearls

- The family should be told that the remaining thumb will always be smaller than the one on the opposite side, because all the material that was supposed to make one thumb has been divided and shared by two thumbs.
- The key maneuvers for this operation are (1) shaving of the metacarpal head, (2) reconstruction of the radial collateral ligament, and (3) resuspension of the abductor pollicis brevis muscle.
- This operation includes an anatomic dissection to ensure that the flexor and extensor tendons are as straight as possible. Even with the best surgical care, the thumb probably will be deviated.

Pitfalls

Pitfalls are related to not performing the maneuvers described previously. If the extra thumb is merely resected, then the patient will have a large metacarpal head with no ability to abduct the thumb and an unstable MCP joint. Communication is essential. The family must be informed and understand that the remaining thumb may remain crooked and will be smaller than the thumb on the other hand.

Classic References

Goldfarb C, Patterson JM, Maender A. Thumb size and appearance following reconstruction of radial polydactyly. J Hand Surg Am 33:1348, 2008.
The authors evaluated thumb size, shape, and appearance after surgical correction of radial polydactyly. They noted that although the patients were very satisfied with the appearance, nail width was reduced and interphalangeal joint angulation was increased.

Ogino T, Ishii S, Takahata S. Long-term results of surgical treatment of thumb polydactyly. J Hand Surg Am 21:478, 1996.
Dr. Ogino has a long experience with polydactyly reconstruction. He presented his series of 107 cases of thumb polydactyly.

23 Thumb Hypoplasia

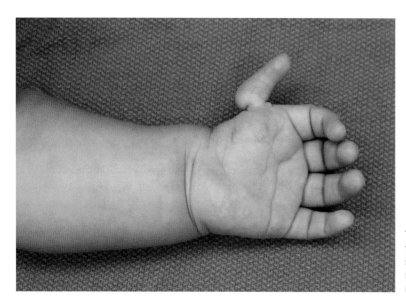

This child has severe hypoplasia of the left thumb and does not use this small vestigial digit. The parents have requested a consultation for surgical reconstruction.

Description of the Problem

The patient has a severe thumb hypoplasia, Blauth type IV, also known as a *pouce flottant.* Because of the severity, the thumb is not functional, and the patient will use his index finger as a thumb in a scissoring position over time. This can be improved with pollicization surgery.

Key Anatomy

The Blauth classification of thumb hypoplasia has five categories. Type I is characterized by minor generalized hypoplasia. Function is normal, and no treatment is necessary. The parents are counseled about the smaller size. Type II involves absence of the intrinsic thenar muscles, first web space narrowing, and instability of the thumb metacarpophalangeal joint with collateral ligament instability. These cases are treated by opposition transfer (usually an abductor digiti minimi muscle transfer), a first web space Z-plasty opening, and collateral ligament reconstruction. The thumb metacarpophalangeal joint instability is the most difficult aspect to treat, because collateral ligament reconstruction usually loosens over time. Manske and McCarroll have subcategorized Blauth type III thumbs into types IIIA and IIIB. Type IIIA characteristics are similar to those of type II, with extrinsic tendon abnormalities but a stable carpometacarpal (CMC) joint. Treatment is similar to treatment for type II thumbs, with the addition of extrinsic tendon realignment or transfer as necessary. Type IIIB is similar to type IIIA but has an unstable CMC joint. Because the CMC joint is unstable, reconstruction of the structures described previously is not effective, and the patient is usually better served with an index pollicization procedure. In type IV, the vestigial floating thumb is best treated with removal and index pollicization. Type V has complete absence of the thumb and is treated with index pollicization. In such advanced cases, index pollicization is favored over toe-to-thumb transfer, because the CMC joint is not stable.

Workup

Patients with congenital absence of the thumb are worked up for systemic syndromic problems, including the following classic syndromes associated with radial deficiency: thrombocytopenia absent radius (TAR syndrome); Fanconi anemia; Holt-Oram syndrome; and vertebral anomalies, anal atresia, cardiac defects, tracheoesophageal fistula and/or esophageal atresia, renal anomalies and limb defects (VACTERL) or vertebral anomalies, anal atresia, tracheoesophageal fistula, and radial anomalies (VATER) syndrome. Genetic counseling with the parents is advised to discuss the possibility of having other children with similar anomalies. An assessment of patients with a small or missing thumb should include a more proximal evaluation of the radius and the associated structures for evidence of radial longitudinal deficiency. Radiographs are obtained to evaluate the underlying radius length and other bony anatomy. Patients are observed during play activities to determine whether the thumb is useful or whether the index finger is being used as a thumb, with a side-to-side pinch. In many cases several visits may be needed for the surgeon, parents, and child to devise a proper reconstructive plan. Index pollicization, if necessary, is a significantly complex procedure that requires all parties to be in agreement.

Treatment

In this child with a type IV floating thumb, the thumb is not reconstructed, because extraordinary lengths would need to be undertaken for an eventual suboptimal result. In some Asian cultures, reconstruction is attempted because of the importance of having five fingers. Generally in the West, the small floating thumb is removed, and the index finger is pollicized to the thumb position at 1 year of age or older. Details of the pollicization procedure are available in the reference.

Alternatives

In this case of a floating thumb, we have discussed that in some Asian cultures, reconstruction has been attempted with fair aesthetic and functional results. In addition, some parents and children choose not to undergo reconstruction. However, in most cases of type IV thumbs, pollicization is a very effective procedure to reposition the index finger into the thumb position as a shorter digit. The index metacarpal is significantly shortened to make this position achievable.

Principles and Clinical Pearls

- The Blauth classification with the Manske and McCarroll revisions is very useful, because it stages the progressive hypoplasia of the thumb and matches each class with a treatment plan.
- In patients with an advanced Blauth classification stage, index pollicization is very worthwhile but technically challenging.
- In all cases of thumb hypoplasia, surgeons must look proximally for evidence of radial longitudinal deficiency. They should evaluate widely for possible underlying syndromes.

Pitfalls

Pitfalls of index pollicization include digital ischemia requiring microsurgical reconstruction, poorly designed skin flaps that result in raw areas requiring skin grafting, and circumferential scar formation. Because the extensor tendon is shortened but the flexor tendon is not, tendon imbalance can occur after pollicization. Opposition transfer as a secondary procedure may be necessary to better position the hand.

Classic Reference

Tonkin MA, Boyce DE, Fleming PP, Filan SL, Vigna N. The results of pollicization for congenital thumb hypoplasia. J Hand Surg Eur Vol 40:620, 2015.
Dr. Tonkin assessed his results from index pollicization, comparing the function of pollicized digits in patients with and without forearm/wrist abnormalities. Results were quite excellent for this series of 35 patients with 42 pollicized index fingers. The range of motion was excellent at the CMC joint.

24 Syndactyly

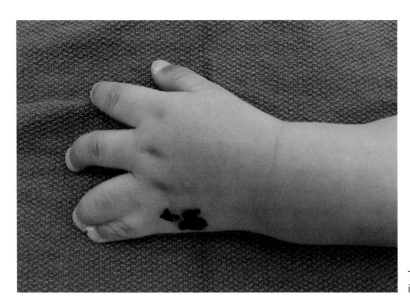

This child has complete syndactyly involving the left ring and small fingers.

Description of the Problem

Syndactyly can be classified as simple or complex. Complex syndactyly involves fusion of the bones distally. Syndactyly is also classified as complete or incomplete. Complete cases have fusion of the fingers all the way to the fingertips. This child has simple complete syndactyly. The fingers are fused at the tips, but the bones are not connected distally.

Key Anatomy

Syndactyly involves the fusion of skin and/or other soft tissue components and possibly bone. A single digital artery can be present between the two fingers. In the border digits, as in this case, the differential length of the two joined fingers may cause deviation over time. Therefore early release of the digits is critical to allow normal longitudinal growth.

Workup

As with any congenital anomaly of the hand, a full genetic workup is required to rule out syndromes and other anomalies. Radiographs are obtained to evaluate the level of fusion and to determine the involvement of bone and cartilage. The hands and feet are examined for other areas of syndactyly. The patient's hand flexion and extension are assessed. In some cases of complex syndactyly, the fingers may have symphalangism with fusion of the joints that prevents flexion.

Treatment

Syndactyly release has several important principles, including elevation of a dorsal flap that will be used to line the web space, zigzag incisions to break up any longitudinal scarring, and coverage of the released areas with full-thickness skin grafts. The dorsal flap and zigzag incisions are carefully designed, and the flaps are elevated. The flap is placed into the web. Lining the web with good dorsal skin is critical to prevent web creep.

The zigzag flaps are inset, and a full-thickness skin graft is harvested from the groin. Careful dissection ensures the digital arteries and vessels are preserved. If the finger toward which a digital artery should be released is not evident, Doppler testing of the opposite side helps to determine whether at least one vessel supplies each finger.

Full-thickness skin grafts should be harvested from as far laterally as possible to prevent the transfer of hair-bearing skin to the hand. Dressings are critical to maintain the web space and to prevent sloughing of the skin grafts.

Alternatives

Many flap design techniques have been described for syndactyly release. Most involve the placement of dorsal skin for the web space. Some authors try to separate the fingers with extensive dissection so that no skin grafting is necessary. Although this is sometimes possible, preservation of the finger width and prevention of necrosis from skin flaps that are too tight are essential. In cases of symphalangism, a longitudinal incision distal to the dorsal flap is reasonable, because zigzag flaps are unnecessary in patients with stiff joints.

Principles and Clinical Pearls

- Digits of unequal length should be released earlier to untether growth.
- The best local skin, which is the dorsal flap, should be reserved for the web space.
- Full-thickness skin grafting should be performed in most cases to prevent tight, thin fingers, which may result from extraordinary efforts to close each finger.

Pitfalls

In the acute period, skin graft loss can result from disruption of the dressings. This can lead to hypertrophic scarring and/or keloid formation. Infection is always a possibility in cases of syndactyly release. Web creep can occur, and revisions may be necessary to widen each web.

Classic References

Kong BY, Baek GH, Gong HS. Treatment of keloid formation following syndactyly division: surgical technique. Hand Surg 17:433, 2012.
The authors focused on cases of keloid formation after syndactyly reconstruction. They presented their experience with methotrexate to reduce re-formation of the keloids.

Tonkin MA. Failure of differentiation part I: syndactyly. Hand Clin 25:171, 2009.
Dr. Tonkin has written this excellent review of his syndactyly release technique.

25 Epidermolysis Bullosa

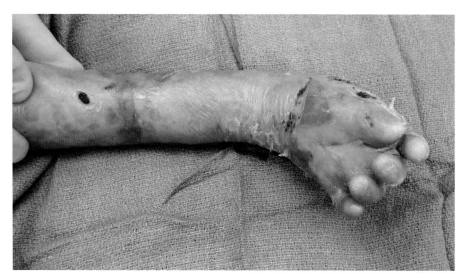

This 5-year-old girl was referred to the hand clinic by a dermatologist. She has severe scarring of her hand with fusion of her fingers. Areas of skin sloughing are present throughout her body.

Description of the Problem

The child has epidermolysis bullosa (EB). This is a group of severe skin conditions caused by deficiency in the ability of the epidermis to anchor to underlying layers. It is a devastating condition, because the skin is very fragile. These patients have difficulties with oral sores, preventing adequate feeding, and extremity problems, including pseudosyndactyly of the fingers.

Key Anatomy

All contact areas of the hand, especially between the fingers, become raw with the simplest activity. This causes healing with scarring. The web spaces fuse together. The thumb web scarring limits any computer activity. Over time, the proximal interphalangeal (PIP) joints develop flexion contractures.

Workup

EB is usually diagnosed by dermatologists. It has three major subtypes of progressive involvement: EB simplex, junctional EB, and dystrophic EB. These categories are based on the level of blistering in the skin. Radiographs are not necessary. The child should undergo careful evaluation by a pediatric anesthesiologist knowledgeable about EB, because it involves the airway and all contact areas.

Treatment

After careful avoidance of all shearing trauma to the skin as the patient is prepared and draped, the hand is "decocooned," meaning the thick layer of dead skin is peeled off from the wrist level to the fingers. The underlying skin seems raw, but it contains enough epidermal elements to undergo reepithelialization. The syndactyly of the web spaces is easily separated by gently teasing the skin apart. No skin flaps are required. The PIP-level flexion contractures are treated by a transverse skin incision and gentle manipulation of the joint to extension. The fingers are pinned in extension. The full-thickness open areas will usually heal in a few weeks. Skin grafts are not used to prevent another area of poor wound healing. Dressings are left intact for 2 to 3 weeks, but the initial dressing change should be performed with the patient under anesthesia.

Alternatives

This treatment has no alternatives. In the future, gene therapy treatment may help to "cure" this devastating disease.

Principles and Clinical Pearls

- Fusion of the fingers in EB is pseudosyndactyly, not true syndactyly; therefore the treatment is simpler.
- The fingers will inevitably re-fuse if daily careful dressings are not performed.
- Perioperative risks are high in these fragile patients.

Pitfalls

Anesthetic risks are high and include airway compromise and skin slough throughout the body. The greatest pitfall is the certainty of recurrence over time.

Classic References

Eismann EA, Lucky AW, Cornwall R. Hand function and quality of life in children with epidermolysis bullosa. Pediatr Dermatol 31:176, 2014.
This recent article from a large children's hospital was the first to document quality of life in relation to hand surgery for EB patients. As expected, recessive dystrophic EB patients reported the worst hand function and quality of life.

Formsma SA, Maathuis CB, Robinson PH, Jonkman MF. Postoperative hand treatment in children with recessive dystrophic epidermolysis bullosa. J Hand Ther 21:80, 2008.
This article in the hand therapy literature described a postoperative treatment program for EB with initial dynamic splinting, followed by static splinting in combination with exercises to maximize outcomes.

Ladd AL, Kibele A, Gibbons S. Surgical treatment and postoperative splinting of recessive dystrophic epidermolysis bullosa. J Hand Surg Am 21:888, 1996.
This classic paper outlined the operative treatment and postoperative care of patients with EB. The steps of "decocooning", syndactyly separation, and contracture release were presented.

26 Constriction Band Syndrome

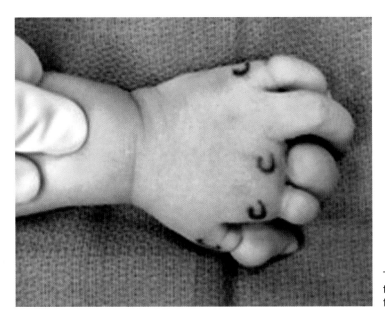

This 10-month-old child is seen preoperatively with a deformity in the thumb, index finger, middle finger, and small finger.

Description of the Problem

The child has constriction band syndrome. This is an in utero condition in which amniotic bands have caused poor circumferential formation of skin, leading to tightness in a bandlike distribution. If the constriction band is very tight, congenital amputation of the fingers may occur. Children with significant congestion and decreased blood flow to the fingers at birth may require emergent surgery. Even if the condition is not emergent, the constriction bands may need to be released to improve appearance and function. The digits distal to the constriction band can be poorly developed, necessitating reconstruction.

Key Anatomy

The key anatomy includes circumferential fibrosis of the skin, leading to poor development distally for all component tissues of the finger. Nerves and arteries may be compressed. Swelling and edema are usually present distal to the constriction band.

Workup

Patients are usually referred to a hand surgeon soon after delivery. On evaluation, if significant arterial ischemia or venous congestion threatens the viability of the digits, emergent surgery may be required to release the band. Usually, however, some flow to and from the digit allows it to survive. In this situation, surgery is delayed until the patient is older and a better anesthetic risk. Patients should undergo a full evaluation for other sites of constriction bands, including the other extremities.

Treatment

The child is deemed a good surgical candidate for general anesthesia. The goal of treatment is to release the tight bands caused by a shortage of skin circumferentially. This is usually achieved with multiple Z-plasties around the digit. Some authors have advocated circumferential Z-plasties; however, most think it is safer to release one side of the digit (dorsal or volar) at a time. In this patient, because the constriction band is very noticeable on the dorsal side, a series of two to three Z-plasties is performed on the dorsal aspect of the thumb, index, middle, and small finger. The tight band itself is excised, and the skin is unfurled proximally and distally, allowing good formation of Z-plasty flaps. If tightness continues in the volar aspect, a secondary series of volar Z-plasties can be performed.

Alternatives

There are no alternative treatments for this condition other than skin grafting and other forms of constriction band release. A patient who loses the digits secondary to constriction band syndrome may be a candidate for other reconstructive procedures, including toe-to-thumb transfer, digital lengthening, and free bone grafts.

Principles and Clinical Pearls

- Constriction band syndrome may be a surgical emergency if the fingers are threatened.
- Surgery consists of releasing the tight band and Z-plasty tissue rearrangement.
- Most surgeons advocate releasing only one side of the digit at a time.

Pitfalls

Pitfalls include having a poor understanding of the urgency of the procedure, leading to loss of the digit. The distal portion of the digit may remain bulbous after treatment because of the chronic edema of the tissue. The zigzag scars can be noticeable as the child grows.

Classic References

Habenicht R, Hülsemann W, Lohmeyer JA, Mann M. Ten-year experience with one-step correction of constriction rings by complete circular resection and linear circumferential skin closure. J Plast Reconstr Aesthet Surg 66:1117, 2013.
The authors presented a large series of cases of constriction rings in the upper and lower extremities. They advocated one-step correction of the constriction rings by complete circular resection and linear circumferential skin closure. This may be more useful in the more proximal areas such as the forearm and lower leg. However, this technique may be less forgiving in the small fingers.

Koskimies E, Syvänen J, Nietosvaara Y, Mäkitie O, Pakkasjärvi N. Congenital constriction band syndrome with limb defects. J Pediatr Orthop 35:100, 2015.
The authors reviewed their registry in Finland on the incidence of constriction band syndrome with limb defects. Constriction band syndrome is rare and makes up 12% of all congenital upper limb defects.

Satake H, Ogino T, Iba K, Watanable T, Eto J. Metacarpal hypoplasia associated with congenital constriction band syndrome. J Hand Surg Am 37:760, 2012.
The authors reviewed the association of congenital constriction band syndrome with distal amputations. They found that metacarpal hypoplasia coexisted with congenital constriction band syndrome in 11 hands in 9 patients. This conflicts with the thought that constriction band syndrome is solely based on constriction with distal amputation. They showed that the cause of these hand anomalies probably is multifactorial.

27 Cleft Hand

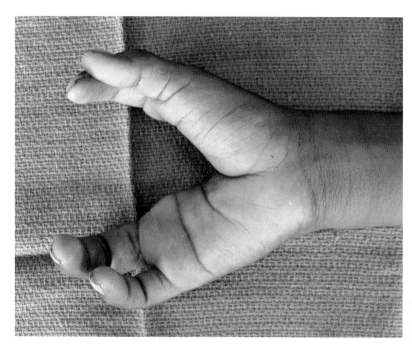

This 6-year-old child is seen in the operating room with a severe cleft hand.

Description of the Problem

Cleft hand involves a significant longitudinal split of the hand along its central access. The missing soft tissue and bone in the central hand creates a very noticeable deformity, including loss of the first web space of the hand. Although the hand may function well with opposition, the appearance usually causes considerable distress for the child and family.

Key Anatomy

In a cleft hand, the index finger is usually radially connected to the thumb, with progressive absence of the first web space. The central portion of the hand has a significant amount of tissue loss, including metacarpal bone and the middle finger. The bony anatomy of the central portion of the hand can be quite abnormal, involving missing metacarpals or a transverse metacarpal. The soft tissue absence results in a cleftlike appearance. Manske has classified cleft hands based on the progressive narrowing of the thumb web. Type I has a normal web, type II has a narrowed web, type III has a syndactylized web, type IV has a merged first web, and type V has an absent first web.

Workup

When a child presents to the Pediatric Hand clinic, careful evaluation of the function of the hand is essential. The ability of the thumb and index finger to oppose to the ulnar side of the digits is assessed. Flexion and extension of the fingers is documented. Radiographs are critical for evaluation of the underlying bony anatomy. The child and family must be counseled that although the appearance may improve, the function will probably stay the same or even decrease as the child adjusts to this new position of the index finger. These abnormalities are usually bilateral and may involve the feet. The other extremities should be evaluated.

Treatment

Because of the appearance of the hand, the child and family may seek reconstructive treatment. In all operations, the index finger is released from the thumb and returned to its position along the ulnar side of the hand to re-create a new first web space. Depending on the bony anatomy, the transverse metacarpal or extra metacarpals may need to be excised. The index finger distal metacarpal is usually placed on top of a remaining ulnar-sided metacarpal and fixed with K-wires. Release of the index finger from the thumb may require syndactyly release distally. Careful evaluation of the nerve and arterial anatomy is critical for successful release the index finger from the thumb. Most of the debate on surgical techniques involves how to rearrange the skin to re-create a first web space. The classic procedure is the Snow-Littler procedure. A dorsal flap is raised that extends to the volar side, lifting a large flap that will be transposed to the index thumb web once the index finger is returned to its ulnar-sided position.

Alternatives

Miura and Upton have described alternative techniques; the references are cited below. Another alternative is to not proceed with an operation. Children who present at a later age may have adapted to this hand position and have good function. Most of the alternatives are related to the various skin flaps that can be used, as described previously.

Principles and Clinical Pearls

- Although the child presented in this case may be quite functional without surgery, the appearance causes distress and concern to the patient and family.
- Surgical treatment goals include a stable yet mobile thumb, transposition of the index finger to the ulnar side of the hand, a well-developed first web space, and improved appearance.
- Skin flaps should be carefully designed to minimize necrosis.

Pitfalls

This is a technically difficult operation with possible pitfalls, including devascularization of the thumb or index finger during mobilization, malrotation of the index ray after transposition, and flap loss of the tissue reconstructing the first web space. Careful microsurgical dissection and tissue handling are critical to minimize these complications.

Classic References

Aleem AW, Wall LB, Manske MC, Calhoun V, Goldfarb CA. The transverse bone in cleft hand: a case cohort analysis of outcome after surgical reconstruction. J Hand Surg Am 39:226, 2014.
Dr. Goldfarb, following in the practice of Dr. Paul Manske, focused on the presence of a transverse bone in the cleft hand. The transverse bone was not associated with worse outcomes after reconstruction. As Dr. Manske has pointed out, the amount of narrowing of the thumb web space is most critical for functional outcomes.

Miura T, Komada T. Simple method for reconstruction of the cleft hand with an adducted thumb. Plast Reconstr Surg 64:65, 1979.
Miura proposed a modified approach to skin flap rearrangement that differed from the Snow-Littler flap by creating a smaller first web space flap. This was intended to limit the dissection of a large flap and the resulting tissue necrosis.

Upton J, Taghinia AH. Correction of the typical cleft hand. J Hand Surg Am 35:480, 2010.
In this surgical technique paper, Upton and Taghinia nicely reviewed all aspects of the operation, including the realignment of the index ray and a simpler flap elevation to limit tissue necrosis.

28 Apert Hand

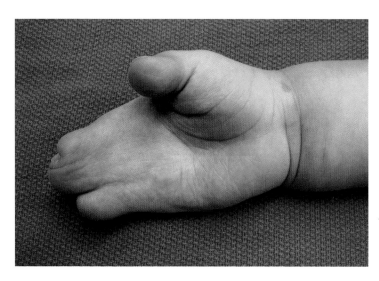

This 9-month-old girl is seen in the pediatric hand clinic with fusion of the fingers of her bilateral hands. Her fingers are stiff. She also has craniofacial abnormalities.

Description of the Problem

Based on the combination of craniofacial abnormalities and complex syndactyly, the child has Apert acrocephalosyndactyly syndrome. This is a fairly rare congenital disorder with craniosynostosis (premature fusion of the skull bones), midface hypoplasia, and bilateral syndactyly of the hands and feet.

Key Anatomy

Characteristic hand abnormalities include a short, deviated thumb with radial clinodactyly; involvement of the first web space with varying degrees of syndactyly between the thumb and index finger; complex syndactyly between the index, middle, and ring fingers typically at the level of the distal interphalangeal joints or beyond; and variable degrees of syndactyly between the ring and small finger. Upton has classified the Apert hand into three types. Type I hands, or "spade" hands, are defined by a complex syndactyly between the index, middle, and ring finger and a simple syndactyly between the ring and small finger. The thumb and index finger are separated, but the first web space may be shallow. Type II hands, or "spoon"/"mitten" hands, are defined by the features of type I hands and an additional partial or complete simple syndactyly between the thumb and index finger and a more complete simple syndactyly between the ring and small finger. Type III hands, or "rosebud" hands, have complex syndactyly between the thumb, index, middle, and ring finger and a complete simple syndactyly between the ring and small finger. The type III deformity is extremely complex and difficult to separate into five digits.

Symphalangism of the digits is an important observation indicating that the proximal and distal interphalangeal joints are not well developed. The fingers remain in an extended position and will not flex actively or passively.

Workup

Apert syndrome is diagnosed based on patient history and physical examination. Radiographs are necessary to assess the amount of bone fusion distally and to show the parents that the proximal and distal interphalangeal joints are not well developed. The patient should undergo a genetic evaluation. The condition can be inherited in an autosomal dominant pattern, but de novo mutations of paternal origin are the most common cause. Ninety-eight percent of cases are caused by missense substitutions in the fibroblast growth factor receptor 2 (FGFR2) gene.

The child should be screened for any risks related to general anesthesia. Congenital heart anomalies must be ruled out. Because of the midface hypoplasia, the airway is narrowed. This requires special attention during intubation and extubation.

Treatment

Reconstruction of the hand involves a series of staged procedures that are performed with the goals of minimizing the number of procedures, maximizing the functional outcome of the hand, and providing a favorable appearance. The technical goals for reconstruction of an Apert hand address syndactyly, thumb radial deviation, and further revisions.

Syndactyly release in patients with Apert syndrome is unique, because the fingers have some degree of symphalangism, with resultant stiff joints that will not deviate with scarring of the skin incisions. After a dorsal flap is raised to reconstruct the web space, straight-line syndactyly release incisions can be made. These prevent the zigzag incisions from extending onto the dorsal and volar surface of the fingers and allow the application of one piece of skin graft to each side of the finger. Because many syndactylized fingers in Apert syndrome are complex (involving bone at the tip), two specific operative maneuvers are critical. Zigzig fingertip flaps, attributed to Buck-Gramcko, are useful for re-creating the nail folds. Intraoperative fluoroscopy is used to visualize the bony fusion before osteotomy. A fine-gauge needle is placed slightly off center to the proposed longitudinal osteotomy, and the osteotome is slid on top of the needle to allow precise sectioning of the bone.

The preferred management of this first web space includes a four-flap Z-plasty, a dorsal rotation-advancement flap for more severe syndactylies, or full-thickness skin grafting for severe type III hands in which local flaps do not provide adequate soft tissue coverage.

The thumb clinodactyly is corrected by a careful osteotomy of the delta phalanx and opening of the wedge osteotomy. The thumb may remain shortened and require secondary bone grafting or distraction osteogenesis when the patient is older.

Alternatives

The need for syndactyly release is without controversy. However, the number of procedures needed is debatable. Some have advocated complete release of all digits at one operation or simultaneous bilateral procedures, but this is unnecessarily complicated for both the surgeon and the parents. For the most complex, type III hand, some surgeons prefer to have three fingers and one thumb as a result. However, it is reasonable to attempt to separate the digits into a five-fingered hand with the understanding that this may not be possible.

Principles and Clinical Pearls

- Complex syndactylies can be released with dorsal flaps for the web, straight-line incisions in the midline, and zigzag incisions at the fingertips.
- Parents should be advised that the fingers will remain stiff after syndactyly release.
- Surgeons should be aware of the anesthetic risks involved in this syndrome.

Pitfalls

The major pitfall is skin graft loss and the need for revision surgery. Web space creep and recurrence of syndactyly is reported in most authors' series. Therefore the recommended duration for postoperative splinting ranges from 2 to 3 weeks. The goal for this prolonged period of initial dressing is to minimize motion and friction at the sites of the grafts and flaps.

Classic References

Chang J, Danton TK, Ladd AL, Hentz VR. Reconstruction of the hand in Apert syndrome: a simplified approach. Plast Reconstr Surg 109:465, 2002.

The sequence of operations was outlined in this retrospective review. Complete reconstruction was performed in 3- to 4-staged operations.

Oishi SN, Ezaki M. Reconstruction of the thumb in Apert syndrome. Tech Hand Up Extrem Surg14:100, 2010.

Optimal reconstruction of the thumb is extremely difficult because the digit is short and deviated. These experts presented useful technical tips, including a unique V-to-Y, Y-to-V flap design.

Upton J. Apert syndrome. Classification and pathologic anatomy of limb anomalies. Clin Plast Surg 18:321, 1991.

This article established the widely accepted Upton classification scheme of type I to III Apert hands.

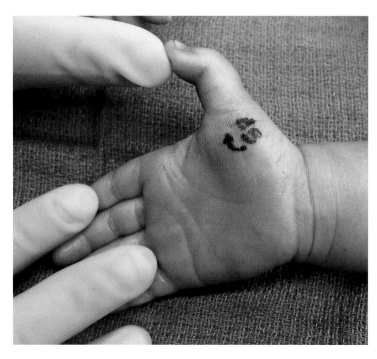

This 1-year-old girl is seen in consultation after her parents noticed that she could not straighten the tip of her right thumb. The parents do not recall any previous trauma. This condition is not painful to the child.

Description of the Problem

The child has a trigger thumb with swelling of the flexor pollicis longus tendon that prevents easy gliding underneath the A1 pulley of the thumb. This may not be noticed for some time, because it is usually not painful and the child quietly adapts. Occasionally, it can be painful if the thumb interphalangeal joint is forced into a straight position. The reason some children develop swelling of the tendon is not known.

Key Anatomy

The critical anatomic concept of trigger thumb is that the flexor pollicis longus is swollen exactly at a site just proximal to the overlying A1 pulley of the thumb. This nodule, known as *Notta's node,* is integral to the tendon itself and is not caused by swelling of the tenosynovium, as in adult trigger thumb. With fixed flexion of the interphalangeal joint, the metacarpophalangeal joint develops compensatory hyperextension. Early surgery may prevent continued hyperextension laxity at the metacarpophalangeal joint.

Workup

Trigger thumb is diagnosed with patient history and physical examination. Radiographs are not necessary, but many parents provide them after initial consultation with pediatricians who may have been concerned with a dislocation. A physical examination reveals a lump at the A1 pulley region, inability to actively and passively extend fully at the interphalangeal joint, and compensatory hyperextension at the metacarpophalangeal joint. Patients should be screened for risks related to general anesthesia.

Treatment

Few case series have reported resolution of triggering over time. However, the time to resolution may be years, and the child may develop hyperextension of the metacarpophalangeal joint if the triggering is not corrected. In most cases, the parents are offered a period of observation before surgery. In our experience, patients most often proceed to surgery. Patients are usually young children; therefore they need to undergo general anesthesia. The thumb contracture is confirmed, and a transverse incision is made in the A1 pulley crease. Careful attention is paid to the radial digital nerve, which crosses over the incision. It is subcutaneous. Scissors are used to gently spread to the level of the A1 pulley. In children, the flexor tendon sheath is very thin; therefore care is taken to incise the sheath and A1 pulley without damaging the underlying flexor tendon. Once the A1 pulley is released, the thumb should easily be extended at the interphalangeal joint. The more distal, oblique pulley is preserved to prevent bow-stringing of the tendon. Full release of the enlarged tendon is confirmed on inspection. The incision is closed with interrupted absorbable sutures. Dressings are critical to prevent the child from disrupting the skin closure.

Alternatives

Some patients have a history of antecedent trauma. Surgery can be delayed a few months to allow swelling to diminish in the hope that the tendon will easily glide again. Corticosteroid injections will not be successful, because the pathophysiology is not tenosynovial swelling; it is an enlarged nodule within the tendon. Surgery is the preferred treatment.

Principles and Clinical Pearls

- This classic presentation may be misdiagnosed as a thumb dislocation.
- Surgery is straightforward and prevents the long-term problems of fixed interphalangeal joint flexion and metacarpophalangeal joint hyperextension.
- The surgeon should understand that trigger finger in digits other than the thumb is not as simple as an enlarged Notta's node but is probably the result of an abnormal insertion of the flexor digitorum superficialis tendon. Therefore surgery for trigger finger (not trigger thumb) requires an extended incision and tendon exploration.

Pitfalls

Incomplete release, overrelease, and digital nerve injury are the avoidable complications. The wound needs to be protected to prevent the child from picking at and scratching the incision.

Classic References

Baek GH, Lee HJ. The natural history of pediatric trigger thumb: a study with minimum of five years follow-up. Clin Orthop Surg 3:157, 2011.
In this series from Korea, the authors prospectively followed 87 thumbs in 67 patients with pediatric trigger thumb. The patients did not receive any treatment, including passive stretching, splinting, or surgery. The trigger thumbs resolved spontaneously in 75% of patients without treatment. However, the average time to resolution was 49 months.

Marek DJ, Fitoussi F, Bohn DC, Van Heest AE. Surgical release of the pediatric trigger thumb. J Hand Surg Am 36:647, 2011.
The authors focused on the decision-making process for surgical release of pediatric trigger thumb. A retrospective review of 217 cases showed no major complications and resolution of contracture in all patients. The authors also surveyed pediatric hand surgeons, and 85% advocated surgical release.

Shah AS, Bae DS. Management of pediatric trigger thumb and trigger finger. J Am Acad Orthop Surg 20:206, 2012.
This comprehensive review discussed the nonsurgical treatment and the surgical technique of trigger thumb release. The authors highlighted the important differences between trigger thumb and trigger finger.

Contractures

30 Spastic Hand and Wrist Contracture

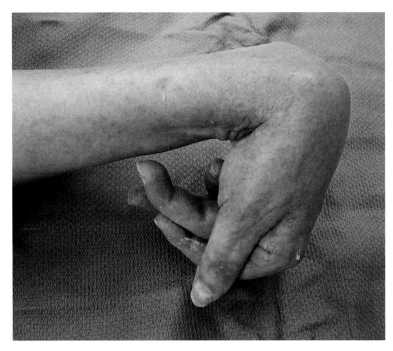

This nursing home patient has a severe contracture of the left wrist and hand. His caretakers find it difficult to provide good hygiene. The nails dig into his palm and cause ulcerations.

Description of the Problem

The patient has a severe hand and wrist contracture after a stroke. The muscles have contracted, leading to severe flexion contractures. This has prevented appropriate hygiene.

Key Anatomy

In this case, the poststroke contracture of the flexor muscles has caused a severe contracture. The flexor muscle tendon units are much stronger than those on the extensor side; therefore they overpower the extensor tendons. This is true of the wrist flexors and the finger flexors.

Workup

The cause of the hand contracture should be determined. In severe contractures, possible causes include cerebral palsy in children, a history of direct hand trauma, compartment syndrome, and poststroke contracture. Patients' medical conditions should be thoroughly understood to rule out anesthetic risks. Before patients and parents provide consent, they should be carefully informed of possible decreased function as a result of placing the hand and fingers in a better position. In the preoperative evaluation, assessment of the level of active flexion in the fingers is critical. In patients with some degree of active flexion, preservation of the motion may be attempted.

Treatment

The initial treatment consists of passive stretching and splinting. Botulinum toxin is sometimes given; however, the contracture usually is severe and fixed in postischemic stroke patients.

The initial surgical treatments are related to extending the flexor tendon unit. A flexor pronator slide may be attempted to release the origin of the flexor pronator mass, allowing it to be positioned more distally. Progressively more involved procedures include fractional lengthening of the flexor tendons, release of the wrist flexors, step-cut lengthening of the flexor tendons, and superficialis to profundus transfer. In a superficialis to profundus transfer, the flexor digitorum superficialis tendons are transected distally, and the flexor digitorum profundus tendons are transected proximally. They are then coapted, allowing one flexor tendon unit to preserve some flexion to the fingers. Last, if the fingers are completely nonfunctional, then a complete tenotomy of all the flexor tendons may be possible to better position the severely contracted hand. Skin deficits should be considered. The hand is splinted with the wrist and fingers extended to prevent recontracture.

Alternatives

If significant contracture persists, alternative treatments include a proximal-row carpectomy to shorten the length of the wrist or wrist fusion. Both procedures require extensive capsulotomy of the wrist joint.

Principles and Clinical Pearls

- Surgeons should determine the cause of a hand contracture to assess preoperative risks.
- Once a patient is confirmed to have flexor function, a procedure such as a flexor pronator slide, fractional lengthening, step-cut lengthening, or a superficialis to profundus transfer should be attempted to preserve some active flexion.
- Postoperative splinting is critical to maintain an acceptable hand and wrist position.

Pitfalls

The greatest pitfall is to underestimate the amount of release that will be required to place the hand in a better position. Surgeons should be prepared to perform progressive procedures, as listed previously. These patients may have severe medical risks, precluding surgery. Understanding the patient and family expectations is essential.

Classic References

Malizos KN, Liantsis AK, Varitimidis SE, Dailiana ZH, Rigopoulos NS. Functional gains after surgical procedures in spastic upper extremity: a comparative study between children and adults. J Pediatr Orthop B 19:446, 2010.
This interesting paper compared spasticity secondary to cerebral palsy in children and adults. As expected, functional gains were better in children; therefore the authors suggested early intervention.

Rosales RL, Kong KH, Goh KJ, Kumthornthip W, Mok VC, Delgado-De Los Santos MM, Chua KS, Abdullah SJ, Zakine B, Maisonobe P, Magis A, Wong KS. Botulinum toxin injection for hypertonicity of the upper extremity within 12 weeks after stroke: a randomized controlled trial. Neurorehabil Neural Repair 26:812, 2012.
In the early treatment of poststroke spasticity, botulinum toxin is an alternative. The authors presented a series of 163 patients who underwent botulinum neurotoxin treatment. They found good results in conjunction with rehabilitation therapy in patients with mild to moderate hypertonicity. Results were best when this was given soon after the stroke.

31 Stiff Finger in Extension

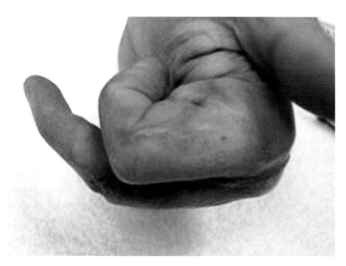

This 33-year-old woman presents with a stiff index finger after closed reduction and percutaneous pinning of a fracture of the proximal phalangeal shaft. Postoperatively the finger was immobilized for 3 weeks with the fingers in the safe position (the metacarpophalangeal joints flexed 70 degrees and the interphalangeal joints extended fully). The patient then started therapy with early passive and active motion. After tenderness at the fracture site decreased, the pins were removed in the clinic, and she underwent active rehabilitation with intermittent splinting. Although she was able to flex her metacarpophalangeal joint fully, she had a limited ability to flex her proximal interphalangeal (PIP) joint actively and passively to 40 degrees. Active motion at the distal interphalangeal joint was acceptable. She has been attending biweekly hand therapy for 3 months, with no progress in her passive or active motion.

Description of the Problem

Fingers that cannot be flexed passively are unable to flex actively. This is a result of dorsal extensor adhesions, dorsal PIP capsular contracture, and contracture and loss of compliance of the collateral ligaments. In some cases, malreduction of proximal phalanx fractures with a resultant prominent volar spike present on lateral plain radiographs can limit passive and active digital flexion and cause the finger to be stiff in extension. In a similar fashion, arthrofibrosis after articular trauma can limit passive and active flexion. Any attempt to correct the lack of passive flexion without correcting extraarticular bony malalignment or intraarticular fibrosis will probably result in incomplete correction.

Key Anatomy

The PIP joint is surrounded by soft tissue structures that serve to guide and constrain its motion. The volar plate attaches the base of the middle phalanx to the distal volar shaft of the proximal phalanx and restricts hyperextension. The collateral ligaments attach the radial and ulnar recesses of the head of the proximal phalanx to the radial and ulnar aspects of the base of the middle phalanx, and the accessory collateral ligaments attach the volar plate to these same recesses. The central slip of the long extensor tendon inserts onto the tubercle of the dorsal base of the middle phalanx. The conjoined lateral bands traverse the PIP joint just dorsal to its axis of rotation and are secured in this position by the triangular ligament distally (restraining volar translation) and the transverse retinacular ligament (restraining dorsal translation). The long extensor tendon sends fibers to the conjoined lateral bands proximal to the PIP joint, which are located adjacent to the proximal phalangeal shaft. All of these soft tissue structures can lose compliance and become adherent to the bone of the proximal phalanx after trauma or fixation.

Workup

PA, lateral, and oblique radiographs are obtained to rule out abnormality or incongruity in the proximal phalanx or the PIP joint. If an intraarticular osteotomy of the PIP joint is thought to have potential value, a CT scan can be obtained to more thoroughly evaluate the joint surface.

Treatment

Once bony healing has occurred and bony or articular abnormalities or incongruities are addressed, therapy can be attempted by active, active-assist, passive, and dynamic passive modalities. If these do not lead to resolution of the stiffness, a dorsal surgical release of the affected tissues is carried out. The long extensor tendon adhesions are freed over the proximal phalanx and the PIP joint dorsally, and the dorsal PIP capsule is released. Collateral ligament recession can then be performed from a dorsal approach, and passive PIP joint flexion can be carried out to evaluate the success of the release. If these releases are performed with the patient under a local anesthetic, then active flexion of the finger is tested when the patient is awake. Otherwise, an incision can be made over the A1 pulley and the flexor checked to evaluate the degree of active flexion to expect after a dorsal release. Extensive releases are not done simultaneously on the dorsal and the volar sides of the finger. This causes pain and swelling that interfere with postoperative therapy.

Alternatives

If the stiffness is painless and the patient can tolerate the degree of stiffness (especially on the radial side of the hand), then nonoperative treatment might be favored.

Principles and Clinical Pearls

- An extensive dorsal release restores passive flexion but does not restore active extension.
- Gains made during a surgical release with the patient under general anesthesia and confirmed by wide-awake flexion or by a flexor check at the level of the A1 pulley will frequently be reduced somewhat during the postoperative period. Patients should be counseled to expect only approximately a 50% improvement (an empiric value) at the final evaluation.

Pitfalls

An inability to extend the PIP joint fully may be a result of an extensive dorsal release, as described. Overzealous hand therapy can stretch the thin extensor tendon, leading to extensor lag after the joint is released.

Classic Reference

Creighton JJ Jr, Steichen JB. Complications in phalangeal and metacarpal fracture management. Results of extensor tenolysis. Hand Clin 10:111, 1994.
This classic manuscript related what might reasonably be expected after surgical tenolysis on the dorsum of the finger.

32 Stiff Finger in Flexion

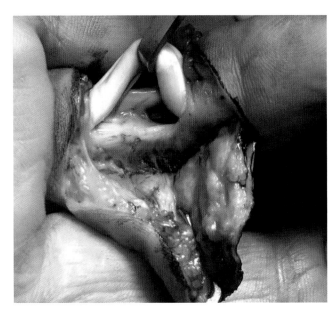

This 46-year-old man developed a progressive flexion deformity of his middle finger proximal interphalangeal (PIP) joint after jamming it while playing flag football. He had immediate pain and swelling after the injury, and he did not seek medical attention. After 3 months, he noticed that he could not extend his PIP joint fully, and after 5 months, he was unable to extend the PIP joint past 90 degrees of flexion. His metacarpophalangeal and distal interphalangeal (DIP) joints remained fully mobile and supple, and he was able to make a fist at full strength. A volar release was planned. After a Bruner-type incision was made and the flexor tendon sheath released, two large, tight, opalescent longitudinally-oriented bands of tissue were observed.

Description of the Problem

The patient has a severe pseudo-boutonnière deformity. This is synonymous with a fixed flexion contracture of the PIP joint. It differs from a boutonnière deformity, which is a hyperextension deformity of the DIP joint with resultant limited full flexion of the DIP joint.

Key Anatomy

A pseudo-boutonnière deformity refers to PIP joint flexion without DIP joint hyperextension. The mechanism causing the deformity is a hyperextension of the PIP joint, leading to volar plate and accessory collateral ligament injury and scarring over the volar aspect of the PIP joints. The normal check ligaments enlarge, contract longitudinally, and cause a fixed deformity of the PIP joint. In this pathologic state, they are referred to as checkrein ligaments.

Workup

Closed injuries of the PIP joint should be evaluated with radiographs. Patients with no fracture or dislocation are examined for full active and passive flexion and extension. Additional imaging is not usually required. Patients should be counseled on the need for dedicated hand therapy after the procedure.

Treatment

Pseudo-boutonnière deformity is frequently a delayed diagnosis, with patients presenting for consultation months after the initial injury. The resulting fixed deformity of the PIP joint should first be treated with serial splinting and exercise before surgical release is considered. Often, the deformity can be partially corrected, and surgical treatment is not sought. Surgical correction involves a volar approach through a Bruner-type incision, release of the flexor tendon sheath, and release of the checkrein ligaments (see figure), volar plate, accessory collateral ligaments, and in some cases the collateral ligaments. Transarticular pin placement to hold the PIP joint in full extension may be needed after the surgical correction of severe recalcitrant deformities. The pin can usually be removed once swelling subsides, usually within 3 weeks of surgery.

Alternatives

Nonoperative treatment can be performed with a digital block, passive manipulation, and serial casting; however, injudicious application of this technique can lead to fractures of the proximal phalanx or the middle phalanx. Some surgeons have reported good success using commercially available devices such as the Joint Jack or the Digit Widget.

Principles and Clinical Pearls

- The difference between a boutonnière and a pseudo-boutonnière deformity is that a boutonnière deformity involves a hyperextension deformity of the DIP joint, and a full fist is not possible.
- The key deficit in pseudo-boutonnière deformity is an inability to fully extend the PIP joint, causing functional and aesthetic difficulties. A full fist is possible.
- Early motion is the treatment of choice after PIP joint injuries; however, the patient and surgeon should be vigilant about the development of a fixed flexion deformity of the PIP joint. In this case, extension splinting is performed.

Pitfalls

A pseudo-boutonnière deformity is not a deformity of extensor mechanism imbalance; however, over time, extensor tendon and central slip attenuation may result in an inability to extend the PIP joint actively after a volar release of the contracted tissues. The fixed flexion deformity of the PIP joint tends to recur postoperatively, often to more than half the original angular deformity.

Classic Reference

Watson HK, Light TR, Johnson TR. Checkrein resection for flexion contracture of the middle joint. J Hand Surg Am 4:67, 1979.
This manuscript described the anatomy of the checkrein ligaments and the surgical tactic for correcting fixed flexion deformities of the PIP joint.

33 Camptodactyly

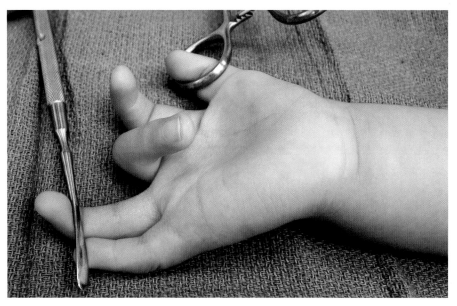

This 4-year-old patient is seen in the operating room with a severe flexion contracture of the right middle finger at the proximal interphalangeal (PIP) joint. The patient has difficulty opening his hand for activities of daily living.

Description of the Problem

The child probably has camptodactyly. This is an idiopathic flexion contracture of the fingers.

Key Anatomy

Many structures have been implicated as the cause of camptodactyly, an isolated congenital flexion deformity of the PIP joint. Skin and subcutaneous tissue, including fascia, the tendon sheath, the insertion of the flexor digitorum superficialis tendon, and the insertion of the lumbricals and interossei, have been described as causing the flexed posture. Over time, the PIP joint itself can remodel. The small finger is most commonly involved, though this can happen in any digit.

Workup

The workup consists of careful evaluation of active and passive motion at the PIP joint. Radiographs are obtained to evaluate the joint for evidence of joint changes and joint fusion. The independent function of the flexor digitorum profundus tendon and the flexor digitorum superficialis tendon are evaluated. The child and parents should be carefully counseled about the limitations of procedures performed to release the joint.

Treatment

The treatment for camptodactyly is controversial. The first line of treatment is passive stretching of the joint and splinting. Authors have shown that passive stretching can improve the flexion deformity in camptodactyly. Surgery should be undertaken only in patients with a severe contraction of greater than 60 degrees that limits function, because results are very unpredictable. It may be possible to fully extend the finger with release of the skin, tendon, and joint; however, this usually results in a stiff finger. Many children are unable to make a full fist after a comprehensive release of camptodactyly. Therefore most authors advocate accepting a slightly flexed position of the PIP joint.

Surgical treatment consists of Bruner incisions in the volar surface of the finger and dissection to release all soft tissue scarring. The insertion of the flexor digitorum superficialis tendon should be carefully examined and possibly released. The volar plate should be elevated and the collateral ligaments released as needed to achieve near or full extension. In some patients, the lumbricals and the lateral bands should be released. A severe shortage of skin may require skin grafting or flap transfer.

Alternatives

The mainstay of treatment for camptodactyly is passive stretching at an early age. The alternatives of surgery and distraction are not favored because of the severe stiffness in extension that may result. Many children and families will accept the flexion deformity when they understand that the child may not be able grasp well with a full fist after surgery.

Principles and Clinical Pearls

- The cause of camptodactyly is unknown, and the deforming forces involve multiple tissues at the level of the PIP joint.
- Early recognition and initiation of a passive stretching and splinting program may improve the flexion deformity to the degree that surgery is not necessary.
- Surgery should be performed only if the flexion contracture is severe (greater than 60 degrees) and the patient and family are thoroughly informed of the likelihood of stiffness of the finger.

Pitfalls

The major pitfall for this operation is stiffness of the finger in extension. The amount of skin, tendon sheath, and tendon requiring release may be so large that after the finger is fully straight in surgery, a full-thickness skin defect results, requiring a cross-finger flap reconstruction. Some patients regret having had the surgery because of these pitfalls.

Classic References

McFarlane RM, Classen DA, Porte AM, Botz JS. The anatomy and treatment of camptodactyly of the small finger. J Hand Surg Am 17:35, 1992.
This classic paper from the University of Western Ontario reviewed the results of 74 consecutive cases for camptodactyly. They implicated an anomalous insertion of the lumbrical muscle as the major cause. The joint contracture was reduced from 49 to 25 degrees. Only 33% of the patients regained full flexion of the small finger.

Rhee SH, Oh WS, Lee HJ, Roh YK, Lee JO, Baek GH. Effect of passive stretching on simple camptodactyly in children younger than three years of age. J Hand Surg Am 35:1768, 2010.
This group from Korea reviewed their results of passive stretching on camptodactyly in children younger than 3 years of age. They showed that passive stretching can greatly improve the flexion deformity. This should be the first line of treatment for camptodactyly.

Smith PJ, Grobbelaar AO. Camptodactyly: a unifying theory and approach to surgical treatment. J Hand Surg Am 23:14, 1998.
This group from London reported on 16 cases of camptodactyly release. They described all volar structures possibly involved in camptodactyly. Because of the complication of stiffness, they concluded that surgery should be reserved for patients with a preoperative PIP contracture of more than 60 degrees.

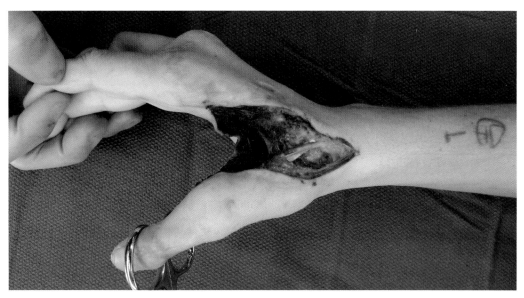

This 24-year-old man had a near amputation of his right hand and has developed a posttraumatic first web space contracture. He is unable to abduct his thumb to grasp a bottle because of the scarred tissue.

Description of the Problem

First web space contractures usually result from trauma with tissue loss or severe scarring. Splinting the thumb in abduction is critical to prevent contracture. The problem is especially debilitating, because the patient can no longer open his hand to grasp large objects such as bottles. Thumb opposition and fine pinch become limited.

Key Anatomy

The supple, pliable skin at a normal first web space allows great freedom of motion for the hand and thumb. The thumb carpometacarpal joint and the mobile skin of the first web are critical for thumb motion. A first web space contracture can include scarred skin, increased fibrous bands, and a tightened adductor pollicis muscle. The dorsal branch of the radial artery is present at the base of the first web. The web space itself has a surprisingly large surface area once fully released.

Workup

First web space contractures are usually posttraumatic; therefore careful review of previous operative notes is essential. Plain radiographs are indicated to assess for arthropathy of the thumb carpometacarpal joint that would prevent full release. The status of the radial artery is examined, because it may be used as an inflow vessel.

Treatment

In the operating room, this patient underwent scar release and release of fibrous bands and a portion of the adductor pollicis muscle to adequately open the first web space. The resulting defect was quite large. It was wide and deep. To provide optimal soft tissue coverage, a lateral arm free flap was harvested from the same arm. The flap's vessels—the posterior radial collateral artery and vein—were anastomosed to the radial artery and cephalic vein. The flap was inset with simple sutures. The donor site was closed primarily; therefore all wounds were on the same extremity.

Alternatives

Common alternative reconstructive options include a reversed posterior intersosseous artery flap, a reversed radial forearm flap, and a variety of free skin or muscle flaps. A pedicled groin flap is an option of last resort. Skin grafts alone are not recommended because of the deep nature of the wound and the likelihood of recontracture.

Principles and Clinical Pearls

- Release of the contracture requires addressing the skin, fascia, and muscle.
- Full release of the first web will result in a defect that is large and deep.
- A lateral arm flap is uniquely suited for first web coverage, because it provides adequate soft tissue fill with minimal donor site morbidity.

Pitfalls

Critical structures at risk in this procedure include the radial artery and the radial digital nerve to the index finger and the ulnar digital nerve to the thumb. Incomplete release of structures will probably lead to recontracture. The size of the defect should not be underestimated. The radial nerve must be identified and protected while a lateral arm flap is harvested.

Classic References

Sauerbier M, Germann G, Giessler GA, Sedigh Salakdeh S, Döll M. The free lateral arm flap—a reliable option for reconstruction of the forearm and hand. Hand (N Y) 7:163, 2012.
In this series, the authors highlighted the use of a lateral arm flap for small and medium-size defects. They discussed the advantages of the flap, including "satisfactory aesthetic appearance, excellent tissue quality, and frequent primary donor site closure."

Windhofer C, Michlits W, Karlbauer A, Papp C. Treatment of segmental bone and soft-tissue defects of the forearm with the free osteocutaneous lateral arm flap. J Trauma 70:1286, 2011.
This paper discussed the possibility of harvesting a portion of the humerus and lateral arm skin for a composite skin-bone flap. This can be used for bony reconstruction in the hand. Surgeons should be very aware of the complications of donor site fracture and radial nerve palsy.

Dupuytren Contracture

35 Dupuytren Contracture

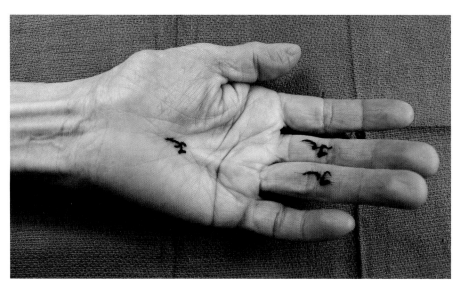

This 52-year-old man is seen in consultation. He has a palpable cord involving his left ring finger and is unable to fully straighten his finger. He states that this has been gradually occurring for the past 7 years. It is not painful, and he is able to make a full fist.

Description of the Problem

The patient has a classic presentation for Dupuytren contracture. This is an abnormal scarring of the fascia and dermis of the hand that causes a tendonlike cord to form, thus pulling the fingers into flexion. It classically begins in the palm and causes flexion of the metacarpophalangeal joints, followed by flexion of the proximal interphalangeal joints. Patients are unable to fully straighten their fingers and have functional problems such as an inability to shake hands and place the hand in a pocket.

Key Anatomy

To understand Dupuytren disease, knowledge of the anatomy of the normal fascia of the palm of the hand and fingers is essential. The fascia is normally thin but strong and separates the tendons and neurovascular bundles into compartments. Fibers are oriented transversely and vertically. The fascia is adherent to the overlying dermis and skin. Once Dupuytren disease begins to form, these normal bands of fascia coalesce into abnormal cords. The pretendinous cord will flex the metacarpophalangeal joints, and as it proceeds distally, will become the central cord that will further flex the proximal interphalangeal joint. The critical anatomic concept of a spiral cord is important. A spiral cord is a coalescing of four normal structures: the spiral band, the lateral digital sheet, Grayson's ligament, and the retrovascular band. Once the spiral cord forms, it will pull the digital neurovascular bundle to the midline of the finger, superficially, and proximally. The thumb may be contracted by an adduction cord.

Workup

Dupuytren contracture is diagnosed with patient history and physical examination. Radiographs are not necessary. A physical examination reveals lumps and pits in the palm in early cases. In more severe cases, cords cause flexion at the metacarpophalangeal and proximal interphalangeal joints, and in the most severe cases, the hand may be in almost a fistlike position. The skin should be carefully assessed for the possible need for a skin graft.

Treatment

The classic treatment for Dupuytren contracture has been regional fasciectomy. However, two alternatives have increased in popularity in recent years and are discussed later. Surgery involves carefully planned incisions to access the diseased cords, while minimizing skin necrosis. Primary cases of Dupuytren surgery usually have enough normal skin to rearrange. However, in secondary cases, a full-thickness skin graft is usually required. Skin flaps are first gently elevated off the diseased cord. At the level of the palm, once the skin is elevated, the cord is exposed. The flexor tendons and neurovascular bundles in the palm are identified and traced distally at the level of the metacarpophalangeal joint and beyond. Surgeons should anticipate that a spiral cord will cause deviation of the neurovascular bundle medially and superficially. Tedious dissection is performed to ensure that the digital nerve and digital artery are safe. It is prudent to make an incision distal to the cord, where the neurovascular bundle is back in a normal position. Thereafter, the neurovascular bundle can be traced in both directions to fully understand its path. The diseased tissue is removed, and the finger is extended into a straight position. Careful palpation should be performed to remove any Dupuytren disease from the vertical fibers in the palm and the skin itself. Once all the disease is removed and the finger is in a straighter position, the tourniquet is let down for hemostasis.

Alternatives

Two excellent alternatives to surgery are available. The first is needle aponeurotomy. In this technique, the palpable cord is perforated with multiple needle holes, and with traction, the cord is broken. The second technique is collagenase injection into the cord at various sites. Over time, this will lyse the cord so that it can be released. Both of these options have a faster return to normal activities, because no incision is needed. However, risks, long-term efficacy, and recurrence rates are not fully determined.

Principles and Clinical Pearls

- Dupuytren disease is a dermal disease. The skin contracture determines the amount of joint contracture.
- Patients need to be carefully counseled about the overwhelming likelihood of recurrence over time. Complete straightening of the finger may not be prudent, because it could prevent active flexion. This is a disease that will manifest over a patient's lifetime.
- Three excellent treatment options for patients with Dupuytren disease are regional fasciectomy, needle aponeurotomy, and collagenase injection. Treatment should be individualized for each patient.

Pitfalls

If the finger remains white with the tourniquet deflated, then the finger is warmed and antispasmodic treatment is initiated. If the finger is still white, a microscope is used to evaluate and possibly repair cut arteries. Along with the dreaded complication of finger ischemia, other serious complications include nerve transection and complex regional pain syndrome. Less serious but more likely complications include skin loss, stiffness, and recurrence.

Classic References

Diaz R, Curtin C. Needle aponeurotomy for the treatment of Dupuytren's disease. Hand Clin 30:33, 2014.
In this review article, the technique of needle aponeurotomy was discussed in detail. Indications and postoperative care were outlined. Links to useful videos showing the technique were provided.

Mickelson DT, Noland SS, Watt AJ, Kollitz KM, Vedder NB, Huang JI. Prospective randomized controlled trial comparing 1- versus 7-day manipulation following collagenase injection for Dupuytren contracture. J Hand Surg 39:1933, 2014.
Collagenase injection is an increasingly common treatment option for Dupuytren contracture release. In the original product design, the patient was to return in 1 day for manipulation. This was inconvenient for the patient and the doctor. In this study, the authors showed that manipulation at 7 days was as effective as manipulation at 1 day. This has led to increased use and patient satisfaction.

Stanbury SJ, Hammert WC. Evidence-based medicine: Dupuytren contracture. J Hand Surg Am 36:2038, 2011.
This short review focused on the best evidence available regarding treatment options for Dupuytren contracture.

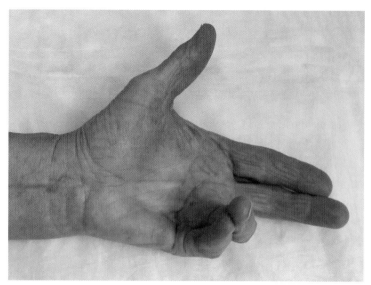

This 71-year-old businessman has recurrent Dupuytren contracture of the small finger 8 years after a volar and digital fasciectomy. He notes progressive loss of passive digital extension over the preceding 18 months, accompanied by the development of a prominent nodule on the ulnar side of the finger, just distal to the metacarpophalangeal flexion crease. He has difficulty placing his hand in his pocket, and in donning gloves. A sensory examination of the finger is normal. A digital Allen test is inconclusive, although review of the previous operative notes does not reveal any vascular injury during the previous surgery.

Description of the Problem

Dupuytren disease can recur after excision or may arise in previously normal areas that have not been excised. Surgeons cannot predict which patients will have recurrence, the parts of the hand that will become symptomatic, or whether further surgical treatment will be needed. In patients with Dupuytren diathesis (an early aggressive form, possibly including the presence of knuckle pads, plantar fibromatosis, and occasionally Peyronie disease), recurrence is thought to be more frequent, more severe, and more extensive. Although nonoperative means such as splinting (static progressive and dynamic), injection of collagenase, and percutaneous needle aponeurotomy have been attempted, none has been shown to prevent or limit the severity or extent of recurrence.

Relevant Anatomy

A common misnomer in the Dupuytren literature is that of the spiral cord. In reality, it is the digital nerve that is pulled proximally, centrally, and superficially by a straight, tight cord of tissue; therefore it may be the digital nerve that is itself spiral and not the cord. Four potential cord types can develop to cause small finger PIP joint contracture: a central cord, a spiral cord, an abductor digiti minimi cord, and an isolated digital cord of the small finger. The path of the ulnar digital nerve of the small finger is slightly different for each of these cord types; however, dissection of the nerve rather than dissection of the cord can decrease the chance of nerve transection. In the finger, the digital artery is deep to the digital nerve. In the small finger, the larger digital artery is usually on the radial side of the finger.

Workup

No imaging workup is needed. A review of the previous operative notes and a digital Allen test or a digital Doppler ultrasonogram will assist in planning for the treatment of vascular insufficiency, should it occur intraoperatively.

Treatment

Surgical treatment depends on the specific goals of the patient. If only digital extension is desired, collagenase injections or a percutaneous needle aponeurotomy (and not an operative procedure) may be indicated. If excision of the diseased volar fascia is needed or requested, options include either a fasciectomy (through a Bruner incision or a linear incision relieved by Z-plasty before closure) or a radical excision of all diseased skin and volar fascia (radical dermofasciectomy). This results in a large wound to be closed by local flaps or skin grafts or by healing through secondary intention. Intraoperatively, the surgeon decides whether to perform a volar plate release of the PIP joint, combined with collateral ligament recessions and release of the contracted fibrous flexor sheath, if present. If this is done, the PIP joint can be temporarily pinned in extension before rehabilitation of the finger flexion arc is attempted.

Alternatives

If the disease severity precludes a repeat excision, the PIP joint can be arthrodesed (combined with as much bony shortening necessary to position the proximal and middle phalanges in an appropriate degree of flexion), or the finger can be amputated.

Principles and Clinical Pearls

- A preoperative discussion of the patient's treatment goals is essential. If only improved digital extension is needed, absent radical excision of the disease, then a nonsurgical approach might be appropriate.
- Dissection of the digital neurovascular bundle should begin proximally in an unaffected area and proceed cautiously through the region where a spiral nerve might be encountered.
- If the finger does not turn pink after release and pinning in extension, the pin should be removed and the digit allowed to flex until perfusion is restored. The finger can be immobilized in this position for a short time before rehabilitation is begun.

Pitfalls

Overly aggressive volar release of the PIP joint can cause a fixed swan-neck deformity. The only treatment for this devastating complication is PIP fusion or amputation.

Classic Reference

Roush TF, Stern PJ. Results following surgery for recurrent Dupuytren's disease. J Hand Surg Am 25:291, 2000.
The authors reported a high degree of patient satisfaction in 18 of 19 patients who had surgery for recurrent disease.

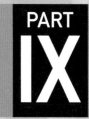

Fractures/Dislocations/
Nonunions/Malunions

37 Radial Head Fracture

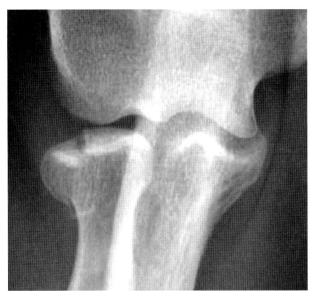

This 37-year-old business executive fell on her outstretched dominant right hand while roller skating for the first time. She felt a pop on the lateral aspect of her elbow, and the area began to swell several moments after the fall. She presented to the emergency department with a painful, swollen elbow held in 60 degrees of flexion. A physical examination revealed point tenderness over the radial head and an inability to actively pronate or supinate the forearm. Passive forearm rotation elicited severe pain over the radial head. Plain radiographs revealed a fracture of the radial head with 2 mm of displacement.

Description of the Problem

Fractures of the radial head occur from a fall onto an outstretched hand. The force of the impact is transmitted through the carpus and radius to the radial articulation with the capitellum. The fracture is classified on the basis of the degree of displacement of the fragment and the degree of comminution of the fracture. Treatment is based on the severity of the fracture and the patient's expectations.

Key Anatomy

The radial head articulates with the capitellum and with the sigmoid notch of the proximal ulna. It is not perfectly circular and has a variable degree of offset from the radial neck and shaft. It has a "safe zone" for the placement of internal fixation that lies in the 90-degree arc subtended by lines drawn proximal from the radial styloid and Lister tubercle. Stability against valgus displacement of the elbow, posterolateral rotatory subluxation of the elbow, and posterior displacement of the elbow is, in part, mediated by the radial head, a prominent secondary stabilizer.

Workup

PA, lateral, and two oblique radiographs are obtained. A concurrent fracture of the coronoid process may indicate a "terrible-triad" injury (consisting of a radial head fracture, a coronoid fracture, and an ulnohumeral dislocation). An early evaluation of whether a mechanical block to forearm rotation exists can inform the plan for operative versus nonoperative care. If the patient cannot tolerate active or passive forearm rotation, and the examiner cannot determine whether a mechanical block exists, an intraarticular injection of lidocaine can be helpful.

Treatment

Nonoperative treatment is the mainstay for all fractures with minimal displacement and full forearm rotation. In some cases, excision of a small fragment of the radial head that mechanically blocks rotation is advisable; however, most of these cases are treated best by internal fixation of the fragment and early motion rehabilitation. More severe fractures such as those that are comminuted and those involving the radial neck may be treated by excision of the radial head and neck and implant arthroplasty. A terrible-triad injury requires the provision of lateral bony stability in the form of either reduction and fixation of the radial head or radial head arthroplasty. Fixation of the coronoid fracture is commonly required.

Alternatives

Early active and passive motion rehabilitation is indicated for minimally displaced fractures or displaced fractures that have no mechanical block to forearm rotation. In fractures that have a mechanical block even after the injection of a local anesthetic into the elbow joint, operative treatment is dependent on the patient's expectation and tolerance for surgical fixation or replacement of the radial head.

Principles and Clinical Pearls

- Minimally displaced fractures are treated by early active and passive motion rehabilitation.
- Arthroplasty of the radial head is indicated if the fracture fragments cannot be reduced or fixed to allow early motion rehabilitation.
- The terrible triad should be appreciated early to initiate appropriate operative intervention.
- The size of a radial head implant arthroplasty should be chosen carefully to prevent "overstuffing" the lateral column. This can lead to difficulty with rehabilitation and can increase the likelihood of radiocapitellar arthritis, which can be disabling.

Pitfalls

Delay in initiation of motion after a fracture can result in elbow and forearm stiffness and can be difficult to remedy by therapy alone. In these cases, dynamic splinting may be needed to regain flexion and extension, and a careful balance between the two is essential to not "rob Peter to pay Paul."

Classic Reference

Pike JM, Athwal GS, Faber KJ, King GJ. Radial head fractures—an update. J Hand Surg Am 34:557, 2009.
This review article discussed current controversies in the treatment of radial head fractures, along with operative and nonoperative treatment.

38 Both-Bone Forearm Fracture

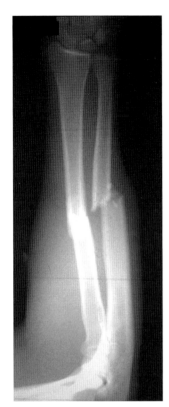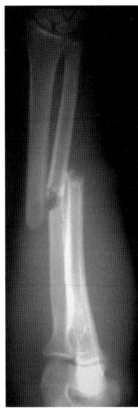

This 21-year-old university student fell on her outstretched left hand while skateboarding. She had immediate pain in her forearm and a substantial deformity on examination. On presentation to the emergency department, other injuries were ruled out by a physical examination and plain radiographs. She was diagnosed with a midshaft both-bone fracture of her forearm, with minimal comminution at the fracture site. Her forearm compartments were soft, and she had intact sensation and motor supply to her hand. Peripheral pulses were normal, and the skin of the forearm was intact. (Image courtesy of William M. Ricci, MD.)

Description of the Problem

Fractures of the radial and ulnar shaft are referred to colloquially as *both-bone fractures.* Although they are not surgical emergencies, several associated complications must be diagnosed early and treated promptly. They include open wounds associated with the fracture and compartment syndrome. The proximal and distal radioulnar joints are evaluated to prevent late presentation of forearm stiffness secondary to malreduction of the joints. Restoration of ulnar length and radial bow is critical to restore forearm rotation and range of motion. Even in open fractures, early internal fixation is essential to maximize functional outcome.

Key Anatomy

The less comminuted bone is reduced and fixed first. The ulna is approached subcutaneously between the flexor carpi ulnaris and the extensor carpi ulnaris muscles. The ulnar plate can be placed deep to the flexor carpi ulnaris muscle to prevent plate irritation. The radius can be approached from the radial neck to the radial styloid through an extensile volar approach described in detail by Henry. Proximally, the interval between the mobile wad and the radial artery is used, and the supinator muscle and the radial and posterior interosseous nerves are retracted radially to expose the proximal shaft. The central portion of the shaft is exposed between the radial artery and the radial nerve. The pronator teres is detached from the point of maximal bow, and the flexor pollicis longus muscle belly is stripped from the radial shaft. Distally, the pronator quadratus is dissected off the insertion on the distal radius. The plate can be placed either volarly or radially. Thompson described an alternate dorsal approach that uses the interval between the extensor digitorum communis and the extensor carpi radialis longus muscle bellies. The radial nerve is identified and protected as it emerges from the distal end of the supinator muscle belly.

Workup

PA and lateral plain radiographs are obtained. A directed examination is needed to identify injury to the median, ulnar, and radial nerves. Compartment pressures are evaluated by objective testing if indicated.

Treatment

Open reduction and internal fixation of both fractures are indicated, followed by early motion therapy for the elbow, forearm, wrist, and hand.

Alternatives

There are no alternative treatments.

Principles and Clinical Pearls

- Patients with both-bone forearm fractures should not be given a nerve block for pain relief, because it masks early signs of compartment syndrome that can occur postoperatively.
- Restoration of the radial bow is the key factor in restoring forearm rotation.
- Although some authors have advocated functional bracing for these injuries, this treatment modality can lead to loss of the radial bow and forearm shortening, with resultant proximal and distal radioulnar joint incongruity. It is not recommended as definitive treatment for this injury.

Pitfalls

Incomplete restoration of the radial bow decreases forearm rotation. Although patients can compensate to some degree for decreased forearm *pronation* by concurrent internal shoulder rotation, the loss of *supination* cannot be relieved by compensatory shoulder external rotation while holding the hand in front of the body.

Classic Reference

Schemitsch EH, Richards RR. The effect of malunion on functional outcome after plate fixation of fractures of both bones of the forearm in adults. J Bone Joint Surg Am 74:1068, 1992.
This classic paper stressed the importance of radial bow restoration to functional outcome after open reduction and internal fixation of both-bone fractures of the forearm.

39 Volar Dislocation of the Distal Radioulnar Joint

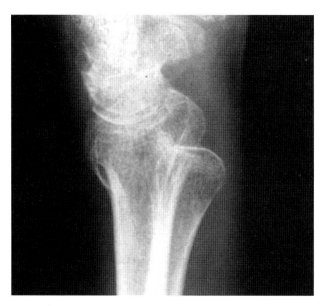

This 23-year-old college student was assaulted while walking home from class. She was carrying her laptop computer in her right hand when an assailant approached her from behind and grabbed the computer. She resisted, and the assailant supinated her forearm forcefully to loosen her grip. She felt a pop along the ulnar side of her wrist, followed by immediate pain. On presentation to the emergency room, she was told that she had no fractures and was sent home. On examination the following week, she held her forearm in full supination and was unable to pronate past 60 degrees of supination. Her ulnar head was prominent volarly and tender to palpation. A sensory examination revealed mildly elevated two-point discrimination in her small finger and the ulnar side of her ring finger. A motor examination was unremarkable, and an Allen test showed intact radial and ulnar circulation. The lateral wrist radiograph is shown.

Description of the Problem

Forceful supination of the hand and forearm can cause the distal radius, carpus, and hand to subluxate dorsally, resulting in distal radioulnar joint (DRUJ) dislocation (a volar dislocation, with the distal ulna anterior to the sigmoid notch of the distal radius). If undiagnosed, the dislocation can become fixed in place, and closed reduction (by dorsally directed pressure on the distal ulna, combined with forearm pronation) is impossible.

Key Anatomy

Soft tissue stabilizers of the DRUJ include the extensor carpi ulnaris tendon and its subsheath, the ulnotriquetral and ulnolunate ligaments (the volar ulnocarpal ligaments), the triangular disc, the volar and dorsal radioulnar ligaments (the superficial and deep components), and the volar and dorsal DRUJ capsule. Following reduction of a volar dislocation, the DRUJ is likely to be more resistant to subluxation if immobilized in pronation. If the distal ulna were dislocated dorsally after an initial injury, the joint would be better immobilized in supination. The soft tissue stabilizers of the joint are critical, because the bony anatomy of the sigmoid notch and ulnar seat (the articular surface of the distal ulna in contact with the distal radius) have substantially different radii of curvature. The sigmoid notch is substantially shallower than the ulnar seat, thereby conferring little or no intrinsic bony stability on the joint.

Workup

PA and lateral plain radiographs of the wrist and an axial CT scan are helpful to evaluate the bony anatomy and the relationship of the distal ulna to the sigmoid notch.

Treatment

Either closed reduction, as described previously, or open reduction through a volar approach (along with a dorsal approach for dorsal DRUJ capsular release as necessary) is performed. Six weeks of immobilization is needed for soft tissue healing. Pinning of the forearm with transosseous K-wires to prevent rotation is optional.

Alternatives

Options for chronic irreducible dislocations include resection of the ulnar seat by a hemiresection (either a matched Watson resection or a Bowers hemiresection) or a complete resection of the ulnar head (Darrach procedure).

Principles and Clinical Pearls

- DRUJ dislocations are most often missed on presentation in the emergency room, because the volar displacement of the distal ulna is not appreciated on lateral plain radiographs.
- Dorsal dislocations of the distal ulna occur with greater frequency than volar dislocations. Closed reduction is often possible, and passive motion therapy to encourage forearm supination, along with volar-directed pressure over the ulnar head, is recommended.

Pitfalls

Focusing on supination (or pronation) of the hand and wrist and not the DRUJ is discouraged, because most or all of the motion will occur through the radiocarpal and midcarpal joints rather than the desired DRUJ. During rehabilitation after a volar DRUJ dislocation, the patient and therapist should manually and directly apply dorsally directed pressure to the distal ulna. Volarly directed pressure to the distal ulna is needed after a dorsal DRUJ dislocation. This therapeutic modality is also performed to treat a DRUJ dorsal capsular contracture and a volar capsular contracture, respectively.

Classic Reference

Kleinman WB. Stability of the distal radioulna joint: biomechanics, pathophysiology, physical diagnosis, and restoration of function what we have learned in 25 years. J Hand Surg Am 32:1086, 2007.
The author summarized current knowledge about the anatomy, pathophysiology, biomechanics, and injuries of the DRUJ and its soft tissue constraints.

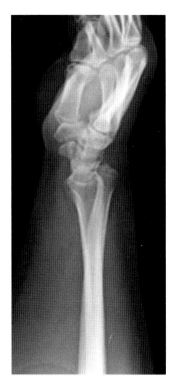 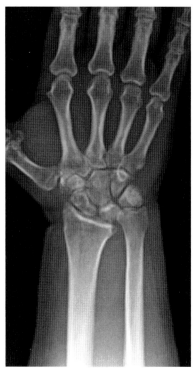

This 28-year-old man fell from a height of 12 feet onto his outstretched dominant right hand. He had immediate pain in his elbow and forearm. On presentation in the emergency department 30 minutes later, a physical examination reveals pain and swelling circumferentially about the elbow, and pain, swelling, and tenderness along the length of his forearm. Examination of his wrist reveals pain and tenderness about the distal ulna and a prominence of the distal ulna that is notably greater than the prominence on the uninjured side. (Image courtesy of Jay Keener, MD.)

Description of the Problem

Fracture of the radial head and neck, combined with an injury to the central band of the interosseous ligament of the forearm, can result in longitudinal instability of the forearm. This injury pattern is associated with an injury to the distal radioulnar joint (DRUJ), causing proximal migration of the radius with respect to the ulna (a so-called Essex-Lopresti lesion). Successful treatment of this lesion surgically requires either stable fixation of the radial head to restore the proper relationship between the sigmoid notch of the distal radius and the ulnar seat or replacement of the radial head with an appropriately sized arthroplasty to restore radial length without overfilling the joint.

Key Anatomy

The central band of the interosseous membrane is wider than 1 cm and attaches proximally on the radial shaft and distally on the ulnar shaft. Because of this direction of travel, application of a force to the radius that serves to drive the radial shaft proximally will cause the ligament to fail in tension. If the bony support of forearm length is lost by fracture of the radial head and neck and the tethering effect of the interosseous membrane is lost as well, there is no constraint to proximal migration of the radius or relative prominence and instability of the distal ulna at the DRUJ.

Workup

PA and lateral plain radiographs of the elbow, forearm, and wrist are needed. Comparison views of the contralateral, uninjured side are obtained to estimate the baseline radioulnar length distally. Stress views (or grip views) can be obtained if a chronic Essex-Lopresti lesion is suspected. MRI can be helpful if a chronic lesion is suspected and reconstruction is being considered.

Treatment

Diagnosis of the lesion as early as possible will alert the surgeon to the necessity of restoring radioulnar length by fixing or replacing the radial head. Although reconstruction of the interosseous membrane has been successful in some authors' hands, salvage of an Essex-Lopresti lesion by late reconstruction has been generally unsatisfactory. Radiocapitellar osteoarthritis can develop with radial head open reduction and internal fixation or with prosthetic replacement arthroplasty, and prominence of the distal ulna may cause ulnar-sided wrist pain if ulnotriquetral abutment occurs or if the DRUJ is incongruent. On a delayed basis, if the elbow is relatively asymptomatic, the ulna can be shortened to relieve impingement of the distal ulna on the ulnar carpus. This is considered only as a temporizing measure while space is adequate for the radius to continue to migrate proximally. Once the proximal radius abuts the capitellum, the migration can no longer proceed, and the distal radioulnar relationship can stabilize.

Alternatives

Early fixation or replacement of the radial head can prevent the lasting effects of interosseous membrane disruption, namely, proximal migration of the radius and disruption of the DRUJ. If this fails or if the injury appears late, then the interosseous membrane can be reconstructed or a one-bone forearm can be created.

Principles and Clinical Pearls

- Maintenance of the radial length and DRUJ congruity is critical for successful early treatment of an Essex-Lopresti lesion.
- If the wrist is symptomatic, an ulnar-shortening osteotomy can provide temporary relief. If the elbow (radiocapitellar joint) is more symptomatic, interposition arthroplasty or a one-bone forearm can provide a stable decompression.

Pitfalls

Playing "catch up" with this pattern of injury once the radius has migrated proximally is fraught with difficulty. The problem has no reliable, consistent solution.

Classic Reference

Marcotte AL, Osterman AL. Longitudinal radioulnar dissociation: identification and treatment of acute and chronic injuries. Hand Clin 23:195, 2007.
The authors outlined the pathologic causes, prevention, and treatment of longitudinal radioulnar dissociation and presented encouraging early results of bone-tendon-bone autograft reconstruction.

41 Distal Radius (Colles) Fracture

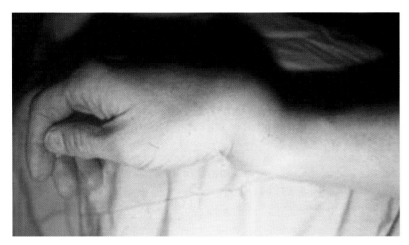

This 47-year-old plaintiff's attorney fell while in the shower and landed on her outstretched right, dominant hand and wrist. She felt immediate pain in the area of her distal radius and noted a substantial dinner-fork deformity. She presented to the emergency department, where a physical examination revealed normal peripheral pulses and a normal sensory and motor examination of the median and ulnar nerves in her hand. A sugar-tong splint was applied. She presents to the office 2 days later for definitive management.

Description of the Problem

A fracture of the distal radius can be caused by a fall onto an outstretched hand. The dorsal cortex of the radial metaphysis fails in compression, resulting in varying degrees of intraarticular and metaphyseal comminution. Reduction is performed, depending on the degree of the deformity (based on measurements of the radial styloid height, the articular surface tilt, radial shortening, and the radial shift), the extent of intraarticular comminution and fragment displacement, and the age and activity demands of the patient. The result of a closed reduction in terms of the measurements mentioned (styloid height, 11 mm; articular surface tilt, less than 5 degrees dorsal; 4 to 6 mm shortening; and less than 2 mm of articular fragment displacement) will inform the surgeon on whether an open reduction and internal fixation would be of value.

Key Anatomy

The tendon of the brachioradialis inserts on the radial aspect of the distal radial metaphysis and epiphysis and subtends the first dorsal compartment. An intact brachioradialis tendon tends to pull the radial styloid fragment proximally and may require operative release if internal fixation and open reduction is deemed necessary. The first, second, third, and fourth dorsal compartments course immediately dorsal to the fracture site. The fifth compartment lies directly over the distal radioulnar joint. The tendons of the flexor digitorum profundus lie immediately volar to the distal radius and the pronator quadratus muscle. The index finger flexor digitorum profundus tendon and flexor pollicis longus tendon course directly over the radial aspect of the volar articular surface. The lunate fossa can extend volarly and provides ulnar-sided support, but the fragment attaches to the short radiolunate ligament and can lead to radiocarpal volar subluxation if it is not fixed.

Workup

PA zero rotation, lateral, and two oblique plain radiographs are obtained to delineate the extraarticular and intraarticular fracture extent. A CT scan can be helpful if a direct articular reduction and internal fixation are considered.

Treatment

There is no universally accepted approach, technique, or implant for the treatment of fractures of the distal radius. Although operative treatment has gained popularity in the past decade (especially the volar surgical approach, combined with volar plating has surged in usage), there is still no satisfactory evidence available that can inform surgeons' choices as to the best technique for reduction and fixation of these fractures. If a volar surgical approach is chosen, then the interval between the radial artery and the flexor carpi radialis tendon is used, with consideration of the potential presence of aberrant branches of the palmar cutaneous branch of the median nerve in the flexor carpi radialis sheath on its deep ulnar aspect. If a dorsal approach is chosen, several intervals can be used, including the interval between the first and second compartment, through the third compartment (with extensor pollicis longus transposition radially), or through the fourth compartment (with subsequent repair of the extensor retinaculum). Internal fixation devices placed volarly can cause volar tendon irritation and rupture, and prominent screw tips can cause dorsal tendon irritation and rupture. Similarly, dorsal internal fixation devices can cause dorsal tendon irritation and rupture (although this is less frequent because the newer plate designs have rounded edges and nonprominent screw heads), and prominent screw tips can cause volar tendon irritation.

Alternatives

Recent studies have informed decision-making with respect to older, less active patients' excellent ability to withstand deformity if treated nonoperatively. Other studies have shown that percutaneous pin fixation of two- or three-part fractures is satisfactory for maintaining reduction until healing has occurred. External fixation or spanning internal plating is useful in severely comminuted fractures.

Principles and Clinical Pearls

- At present, there is little consensus on the benefit of internal fixation in the operative treatment of distal radius fractures.
- Postoperatively, patients should be monitored for the development of complex regional pain syndrome type 2 to ensure prompt surgical treatment, if indicated.
- Although level I evidence supports giving oral vitamin C to help prevent the development of a pain syndrome after a distal radius fracture, this medical protocol is used inconsistently.

Pitfalls

Volar fragment fractures of the lunate fossa can result in volar radiocarpal subluxation or dislocation if not diagnosed and fixed. Median and/or ulnar nerve injury can occur with volar approaches, and radial sensory nerve injury can occur with dorsal approaches. In some patients, a concurrent carpal tunnel release is necessary. In these cases, the volar incision of the release should not cross the wrist flexion crease and should not join with the incision made for fracture fixation. Doing so would risk iatrogenic injury to the palmar cutaneous branch of the median nerve. Finally, bone density testing should accompany treatment of the fracture in patients considered to be at risk for a fragility fracture.

Classic Reference

Apergis E, Darmanis S, Theodoratos G, Maris J. Beware of the ulno-palmar distal radial fragment. J Hand Surg Br 27:139, 2002.
Although not considered a classic of the literature, this paper alerted surgeons to the volar ulnar fragment and the associated pitfalls.

42 Distal Radius Fracture (Smith)

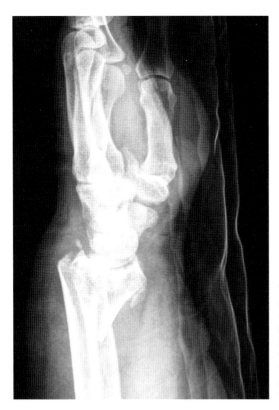

This 19-year-old university student fell outside a bar after a night of drinking. The next morning, his right, nondominant wrist was swollen, painful, and had a noticeable deformity. On presentation to the emergency department, a physical examination reveals a swollen, tender, and ecchymotic distal forearm, with the hand displaced volarly with respect to the long axis of the forearm. The skin is intact, and he has paresthesias without loss of two-point sensation in his median and ulnar nerve distributions. Peripheral pulses are normal. Lateral radiograph is shown.

Description of the Problem

In contradistinction to the common and well-understood Colles-type fracture (see Chapter 41), Smith fractures of the distal radius result from falls onto an outstretched hand with the wrist flexed rather than extended. This causes the distal radial metaphysis to fail in compression on the volar side, with volar displacement of the fracture fragment and the carpus and hand. The fracture line can exit dorsally, proximal to the articular surface (classified as an AO type A fracture), or it can exit through the articular surface and be classified as a volar Barton rather than a Smith fracture.

Key Anatomy

Failure of the volar metaphyseal cortex of the distal radius implies a greater applied force than that causing failure of the dorsal cortex in a Colles fracture. The anatomy of the volar and dorsal distal radial metaphysis and epiphysis is the same; however, surgical treatment of a Smith fracture (or a volar Barton–type fracture) involves a surgical approach volarly and fixation of a volar plate to the radial shaft, with screws placed distally in the metaphyseal fragment to prevent dorsal displacement of the distal fragment. The issues described for volar fixation for Colles-type fractures are applicable for Smith fractures and volar Barton fractures.

Workup

PA zero rotation, lateral, and two oblique plain radiographs are obtained to delineate the extraarticular and intraarticular fracture extent. A CT scan can be helpful if a direct articular reduction and internal fixation is considered or if the precise degree of intraarticular displacement is in question.

Treatment

Open reduction and internal fixation using a plate and screws from the volar side is the standard surgical technique for the treatment of Smith and volar Barton fractures.

Alternatives

In medically unwell patients, these fractures may be managed nonoperatively by closed reduction and cast immobilization; however, the forces acting on the distal fragment that tend to displace the fragment are unlikely to be controlled by this method. Smith fractures that can be reduced closed and pinned percutaneously can be managed in this fashion in selected patients if plating is contraindicated or ill advised.

Principles and Clinical Pearls

- A volar buttress plate is the standard surgical treatment for Smith and volar Barton fractures. Screws should be placed in the metaphyseal fragment to prevent dorsal displacement of the fragment.
- Patients are monitored postoperatively for the development of complex regional pain syndrome type 2 to ensure surgical treatment, if indicated, is performed early in the course of the condition.
- Despite level I evidence supporting treatment with oral vitamin C to prevent the development of a pain syndrome after a distal radius fracture, the protocol is used inconsistently.

Pitfalls

Volar fragment fractures of the lunate fossa can result in volar radiocarpal subluxation or dislocation if not diagnosed and fixed. Median or ulnar nerve injury can occur after volar approaches. Some patients require a concurrent carpal tunnel release. In these cases, the carpal tunnel release incision should not connect with the incision for fracture fixation; therefore the incision for carpal tunnel release should not cross the wrist flexion crease. Doing so would risk iatrogenic injury to the palmar cutaneous branch of the median nerve. Neglecting to place screws in the distal fragment might cause the fracture fragment to become displaced dorsally.

Classic Reference

Nienstedt F. The operative treatment of intraarticular Smith fractures. J Hand Surg Br 24:99, 1999.
In a series of 21 consecutive patients with Smith fractures treated by operative fixation, the best results were in those fixed internally by a volar plate and screws.

43 Distal Radius Fracture Malunion

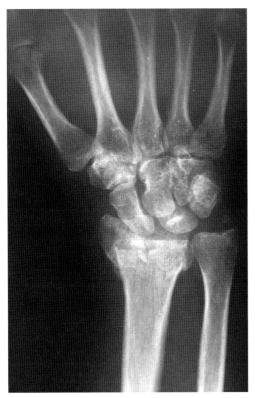

This 40-year-old man fell from a height of 8 feet onto his outstretched right, dominant hand. On presentation to the emergency department, he reported that he had been on a scaffold, felt an immediate crushing retrosternal chest pain, and lost his balance and fell to the ground. He was diagnosed with a fracture of the distal radius and an acute anterior myocardial infarction, with elevation of his ST segments in the precordial leads and T wave inversion. He underwent fracture splinting and emergent stenting of his left anterior descending coronary artery. On the advice of his cardiologist, operative treatment of his distal radius fracture was deferred for 6 months. He presents to the office with an obvious malunion of his distal radius, with ulnar-sided wrist pain and a weakened grip. A physical examination reveals a healed, nontender fracture deformity with noticeable radial deviation of the hand and apex volar angulation at the fracture line. The areas over the ulnar styloid and the midcarpal joint are tender to palpation. A PA radiograph is shown.

Description of the Problem

The degree to which distal radial fracture malunions can help to predict pain and functional loss is a topic of intense debate. Recent studies have shown that in older patients with decreased functional demands, tolerance for deformity is good. In younger patients with a typical apex volar deformity after a Colles-type fracture of the distal radius, midcarpal malalignment may ensue and become symptomatic. Whether correction of the radial deformity by osteotomy will restore midcarpal alignment and capitolunate alignment is unknown. The degree to which the carpus, metacarpus, and hand are deviated radially in these malunions often is the chief reason for presentation and for requesting operative correction of a radial club hand–like deformity. On occasion, radial shortening with concomitant ulnocarpal impaction leads to ulnar-sided wrist pain from abutment of the ulnar pole on the triquetrum, the lunotriquetral ligament, and the lunate.

Key Anatomy

An adaptive, nondissociative carpal instability pattern develops after dorsal malunion of the distal radial articular surface. The lunate remains centered in the dorsally malaligned lunate fossa, and the capitate assumes a position of relative flexion with respect to the lunate (increased capitolunate angle radiographically) in an attempt to keep the metacarpus aligned with the long axis of the forearm. The triangular disc can be eroded if the ulnar shortening is enough to cause ulnolunate or ulnotriquetral abutment. Forearm rotation may be compromised if the distal radioulnar joint is substantially incongruent.

Workup

PA zero rotation, lateral, and two oblique plain radiographs are obtained to quantify the deformity. The contralateral distal radius is imaged to help plan an osteotomy to restore symmetrical alignment. A CT scan with three-dimensional reconstruction is costly and often adds little information essential for preoperative planning.

Treatment

Either a dorsal or a volar approach to the malunited distal radius can be used. The brachioradialis will require release frequently. Either volar fixation or dorsal fixation can be performed. There is no consensus currently on the type of bone graft required to bridge the osseous defect created by the osteotomy. If a volar approach is used, a fixed-angle plate is placed to assist in correction; if a dorsal approach is used, the distal fragment can be levered open using an osteotome and then maintained in the reduced position by structural autograft or allograft. Plate and screw fixation is used for final immobilization to maintain the position during healing. If an intraarticular malalignment is diagnosed and treatment for the malalignment is indicated, a dorsal approach is preferred, with exposure of the articular surface and re-creation of the articular fracture line under direct vision.

Alternatives

In older patients with lower functional demands, deformity (often severe) can be well tolerated.

Principles and Clinical Pearls

- Dorsal exposure with articular visualization is necessary if intraarticular correction is needed.
- The choice of structural or nonstructural autograft or allograft is surgeon dependent. No data confirm the superiority of one graft type over another for healing or maintenance of correction.
- Patients often request operative correction of their deformity for primarily aesthetic reasons.

Pitfalls

In osteopenic bone, a fixed-angle device applied from a volar approach can pull out of the bone during correction. This complication is disastrous and should be prevented by thorough circumferential release of the radial and dorsal soft tissue envelope of the distal fragment. Postoperatively, these patients can have severe circumferential swelling of the wrist and forearm, often with blister formation. This is rarely severe enough to warrant decompression; however, patients should be monitored for median or ulnar nerve compression.

Classic Reference

Fernandez DL. Correction of post-traumatic wrist deformity in adults by osteotomy, bone-grafting, and internal fixation. J Bone Joint Surg Am 64:1164, 1982.
This is the classic manuscript outlining the preoperative planning and surgical technique of distal radius osteotomy after malunion.

Transsscaphoid Perilunate Fracture Dislocation

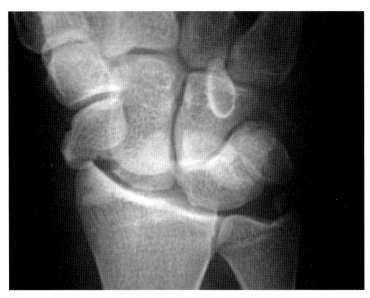

This 26-year-old female motocross racer was thrown from her bike during a race. She ran over a hole while riding in excess of 30 miles per hour and fell onto her outstretched left, dominant hand. She felt immediate pain in her wrist and noticed a pronounced deformity once her gloves were removed. The patient presents to the emergency department, where other injuries are ruled out. She has a noticeable deformity in which her hand is translated dorsally with respect to her wrist and forearm. The area over the dorsum of her wrist and her anatomic snuffbox are tender. Her median and ulnar nerve have intact motor function and two-point discrimination; however, she has tightness and tingling sensations in her median and ulnar sensory distributions. The skin is intact. A PA radiograph of the wrist is shown.

Description of the Problem

Transsscaphoid perilunate fracture dislocations of the wrist are part of the spectrum of perilunate (dissociative proximal carpal row) instabilities. Because the fracture extends through the scaphoid, the dislocation is referred to as *transsscaphoid*. If other fractures are present (which is possible given the direction of the applied force), then the dislocation can be called a *transradial styloid, capitate, triquetrum, and/or ulnar styloid fracture dislocation*. Perilunate dislocations accompanied by any of these fractures are known as *greater arc injuries*, whereas perilunate dislocations not associated with carpal or radioulnar fractures are *lesser arc injuries*. The key components to treatment of these injuries are the diagnosis of the fractures and dislocations, fixation of the fractures where applicable, and reduction and pinning of the dislocations until soft tissue has healed.

Key Anatomy

High-energy deviation and twisting force applied to the radial wrist causes force transmission across the radiocarpal and ulnocarpal joints as well as the carpal bones in a radial to ulnar direction. The most commonly encountered greater arc injury involves avulsion of the extrinsic radiocarpal volar ligaments, fracture of the scaphoid waist, capitolunate dislocation, lunotriquetral ligament tear, and fracture of the ulnar styloid, with a variable degree of damage to the triangular fibrocartilage complex. The dorsal radiocarpal and dorsal intercarpal ligaments are also disrupted. Although the scapholunate ligament is frequently intact in a scaphoid fracture, this is not always the case; often, the proximal scaphoid pole may be devoid of bony or ligamentous attachment. This necessarily causes avascular necrosis of the proximal pole and may affect bony and ligamentous healing adversely.

Workup

PA, lateral, and oblique plain radiographs are obtained. Considerations include the relationship between the proximal scaphoid pole and the radial aspect of the lunate, the relationship between the capitate and the lunate, the relationship between the lunate and the triquetrum, and the presence or absence of radial styloid fractures or other carpal greater arc fractures. A fracture of the capitate waist and inversion of the proximal capitate pole constitute a scaphocapitate syndrome. Open reduction and internal fixation of both the capitate and the scaphoid must proceed urgently.

Treatment

All fractures are treated by open reduction and internal fixation, followed by pinning of all radiocarpal and intercarpal dislocations. All fractures are openly reduced through a dorsal approach. Pins are directed toward the carpus from both radial- and ulnar-sided small incisions near the carpus to minimize the potential for radial sensory or ulnar nerve irritation. Pins are left in place for a minimum of 8 weeks and often longer if pin-site infection does not develop. After the pins are removed, wrist mobility and grip strength are addressed by synergistic grip–range of motion therapy and intermittent splinting. Passive stretching of the wrist to regain motion is not recommended, because it can stress the ligament repairs.

Alternatives

These injuries are not treated nonoperatively. In the hands of especially skilled arthroscopists, they may possibly be treated arthroscopically.

Principles and Clinical Pearls

- Pins placed to maintain reduction of the dislocations are left in place for at least 8 weeks. This length of time is necessary for sufficient soft tissue healing to minimize the possibility of late static carpal instability.
- Small incisions should be made over the radial styloid and the scaphoid radially and over the triquetrum ulnarly to minimize cutaneous nerve irritation or injury.
- These fractures are often fixed with headless compression screws; however, pin fixation is acceptable if the fragments are of insufficient size or quality for internal fixation.

Pitfalls

Malreduction, insufficient time of immobilization, and fracture nonunions can lead to adverse outcomes. Patients are at risk for carpal tunnel syndrome and/or hand and forearm compartment syndrome.

Classic Reference

Forli A, Courvoisier A, Wimsey S, Corcella D, Moutet F. Perilunate dislocations and transscaphoid perilunate fracture-dislocations: a retrospective study with minimum ten-year follow-up. J Hand Surg Am 35:62, 2010.
Eighteen patients were evaluated a minimum of 10 years after injury and treatment. Although radiographic arthritis was common, symptoms were tolerable and functional deficit was "well tolerated."

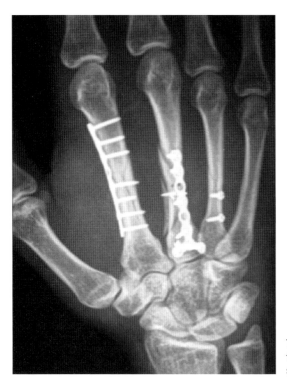

This patient had open reduction and internal fixation for multiple metacarpal fractures. This oblique radiograph is taken soon after the operation.

Description of the Problem

Multiple metacarpal fractures can be treated in a variety of ways. However, open reduction and internal fixation allows earlier return to activities.

Key Anatomy

The alignment of the metacarpal bones is important to understand during open reduction and internal fixation. First, the length of the metacarpals should be established, and the proper rotation should be controlled. The index and middle finger metacarpals are longer than those of the ring finger and small finger. Reestablishment of normal height is important. If a fracture is malaligned and the reduction and fixation is not anatomically correct, then malrotation with scissoring of the fingers can occur. Shortening can lead to loss of the normal contours of the dorsal hand with flexion.

Workup

In any patient with multiple metacarpal fractures, one must presume it is a high-energy injury. Therefore ruling out compartment syndrome of the hand emergently is essential. The surgeon is unlikely to be able to reduce and maintain alignment of the fractures. A sensory and nerve examination should be performed to ensure there is no nerve involvement. Open wounds necessitate earlier operation. In most cases, comprehensive radiographs of the hand are sufficient to diagnose the fracture pattern. In more complex injuries with bony loss, a three-dimensional CT scan may be helpful. Patients should be counseled on the possibility of nonunion, malunion, and stiffness of the hand after surgery.

Treatment

This patient has three metacarpal fractures. Treatment of all fractures may be possible through one longitudinal incision or through two parallel, longitudinal incisions spaced apart to ensure adequate blood supply to the skin between the incisions. The extensor tendons are retracted and protected. The periosteum over each metacarpal is incised sharply and dissected free circumferentially to expose the fracture pattern. Each fracture is unique; therefore understanding the three-dimensional orientation of each one is critical. Fractures are reduced, with careful visualization of the fracture pattern reduction. Fluoroscopy is used to confirm fracture reduction. The most important criterion for successful fracture reduction is passive placement of the hand in a fist without scissoring of the fingers. Each fracture is reduced and fixed individually in sequence. In this example, different fixation methods were used. The index metacarpal had a comminuted fracture with a transverse component; therefore a plate was used. The middle finger metacarpal had a severe comminution with a butterfly fragment that was captured with a cerclage wire, and then a plate was placed with extra holes at the metacarpal base. The ring finger metacarpal fracture was oblique and stabilized with two lag screws. All three fractures were reduced, allowing stable fixation for range of motion. The screw lengths were noted to be adequate and not too long. The periosteum was carefully closed, and the extensor tendons were returned to their appropriate positions. The skin was closed and a volar splint placed.

Alternatives

This patient is unlikely to achieve reduction and stabilization nonoperatively because of the instability across several bones. If only one metacarpal is fractured, often the reduction leads to some degree of stability that can be followed over weeks with serial radiographs to monitor for displacement. K-wires or other interosseous wiring can be used as alternatives. Plates were chosen in this case to allow earlier range of motion therapy.

Principles and Clinical Pearls

- Hand compartment syndrome should be suspected when a high-energy injury has resulted in multiple metacarpal fractures.
- Each fracture has its own personality. One must carefully determine the fracture pattern and the proper reduction.
- The minimal fixation method is chosen that will allow a stable construct in early range of motion therapy, without excessive hardware or dissection.

Pitfalls

Pitfalls include nonunion and malunion with poorly reduced fracture fixation. Extensor tendon scarring and/or rupture can occur. The most common preventable complication is stiffness of the hand. Many novice hand surgeons are afraid to move the hand immediately after fracture fixation. This results in a stiff, poorly functioning hand.

Classic References

Bloom JM, Hammert WC. Evidence-based medicine: metacarpal fractures. Plast Reconstr Surg 133:1252, 2014.
This recent review article was an excellent evidence-based study of metacarpal fractures. It covered the various fixation techniques, ranging from conservative management to internal fixation with plates and screws.

Friedrich JB, Vedder NB. An evidence-based approach to metacarpal fractures. Plast Reconstr Surg 126:2205, 2010.
This was a maintenance-of-certification, evidence-based review article on metacarpal fractures, specifically citing the level of evidence for each paper.

Neumeister MW, Webb K, McKenna K. Non-surgical management of metacarpal fractures. Clin Plast Surg 41:451, 2014.
This paper focused on nonsurgical management of metacarpal fractures. It advocated the most conservative approach that will allow rapid recovery with normal range of motion.

46 Phalanx Fracture

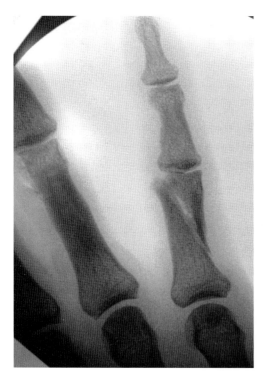

This 31-year-old restaurant server was finger wrestling with another server when he felt a snap in the region of the proximal phalanx of his index finger. He noted immediate deformity, with the index finger deviated radially in the frontal plane. He also noted the finger was rotated in supination. He pulled on the finger almost immediately and was able to realign the finger longitudinally; however, the rotational deformity persisted. On presentation to the emergency department, he had a closed fracture of the proximal phalangeal shaft and a substantial rotational deformity on resting posture and with attempted digital flexion. The PA radiograph shows the fracture.

Description of the Problem

Digital phalanx fractures are the result of either direct or indirect (as in this case) force applied to the finger. The fracture pattern can be transverse (with or without extrusion wedge fragments) or short oblique in the event of a force applied directly, or spiral (with or without additional fracture lines) if the force was applied indirectly. An apex volar deformity can result and lead to an extensor lag at the proximal interphalangeal joint because of altered extensor tendon biomechanics. However, the primary reason for closed reduction with or without surgical fixation is the presence of a rotational deformity made obvious and disabling by digital flexion. The finger can either curl under the adjacent middle finger (as in this case), or the tip can diverge from the middle fingertip when a fist is attempted. This can lead to decreased dexterity, decreased grip strength, and altered fine grasp and pinch activity.

Key Anatomy

The extensor mechanism is relatively shortened with an apex volar angulation. This leads to a lag at the proximal interphalangeal joint and an extension deformity at the distal interphalangeal joint. Incomplete digital extension and an inability to flex the finger pulp to touch grasped objects can result. This pattern of deformity is akin to an imbalance of the extensor mechanism present with boutonnière deformity. The proximal phalanx itself is shrouded dorsally by the long digital extensor and volarly by the fibrous flexor sheath. Radially and ulnarly, the conjoined lateral bands and the transverse retinacular ligaments are adjacent to the phalanx at its midportion, and distally and proximally the sagittal bands are applied to the phalanx closely. With open reduction, all of these retinacular structures risk substantial adhesion formation to the phalanx and to any internal fixation device used for fixation of the fracture.

Workup

PA, lateral, and oblique plain radiographs are obtained. If a displaced articular component is not fully understood on plain radiographs, a CT scan with or without three-dimensional reconstruction can be obtained. Other preoperative observations include the direction and the degree of rotational displacement of the finger and whether rotational alignment is completely normal on the contralateral side.

Treatment

A digital block or a peripheral nerve block is given before a closed reduction. Percutaneous pins can be introduced either in the proximodistal direction or from the radial and/or ulnar sides of the finger to obtain purchase in both main fracture fragments. Pins are left in place until local tenderness at the fracture site cannot be elicited with moderate pressure. Early active and active-assist range of motion can help to preserve suppleness of adjacent joints. After pin removal, active range of motion therapy with or without splinting or buddy taping can hasten motion recovery.

Alternatives

Open reduction and internal fixation using plates and screws can be performed using a dorsal approach (extensor tendon splitting) or a lateral (midaxial) approach. If a midaxial approach is chosen, resection of the distal sagittal band and the transverse retinacular ligament on the side of the implant might decrease adhesion formation and the likelihood of hardware removal and tenolysis.

Principles and Clinical Pearls

- Less is more. If surgical treatment is required, percutaneous fixation is preferred unless internal fixation will allow very early motion rehabilitation without substantial risk of fixation failure.
- All fingers and joints not involved in the trauma or fixation should begin early range of motion therapy.
- The presence of any degree of rotational deformity is not reason enough for surgical reduction. The finger should scissor either radially or ulnarly during flexion to an extent that the surgeon considers unacceptable.

Pitfalls

Open reduction and pin fixation combines adhesion-forming surgery with incomplete stabilization and is to be eschewed. After a phalanx fracture occurs, an underappreciated rotational deformity that has led to a malunited proximal phalanx fracture can be treated by rotational osteotomy through either the metacarpal or the proximal phalanx.

Classic Reference

Eberlin KR, Babushkina A, Neira JR, Mudgal CS. Outcomes of closed reduction and periarticular pinning of base and shaft fractures of the proximal phalanx. J Hand Surg Am 39:1524, 2014.
A retrospective series of 43 patients treated for 50 fractures was reviewed. Results were generally satisfactory after percutaneous periarticular pinning. Time to healing averaged 4 weeks.

47 Proximal Interphalangeal Joint Fracture Dislocation (Dorsal)

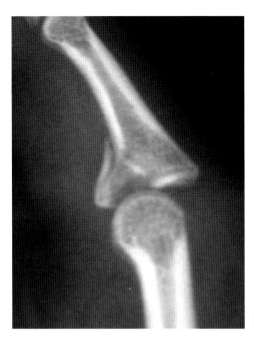

This 25-year-old graduate student jammed his nondominant ring finger while attempting to catch a football. He was unable to flex the finger at the proximal interphalangeal (PIP) joint after the injury, and swelling and bruising became apparent within the hour. He sought emergency care. Lateral view radiograph is shown.

Description of the Problem

Dorsal fracture dislocations of the PIP joint result from an axial load applied to the joint during trauma to the tip of the finger. They are often discounted by the patient as a sprain or a jammed finger, and emergency care is frequently delayed. The volar articular surface of the PIP joint is separated from the rest of the middle phalanx (a partial articular fracture). The joint no longer has the intrinsic stability to remain reduced, which is provided by the articular surface of the proximal aspect of the middle phalanx and the proper and accessory collateral ligaments. Loss of the volar plate and accessory collateral ligament attachment to the middle phalanx, along with volar articular loss, contributes to dorsal instability.

Key Anatomy

Stability of the PIP joint is dependent on an intact middle phalangeal articular surface and intact collateral ligaments and accessory collateral ligaments. The collateral ligaments originate at the center of rotation of the head of the proximal phalanx and insert on the radial and ulnar aspects of the base of the middle phalanx. The accessory collateral ligaments also originate on the proximal phalanx but insert into the distal aspect of the volar plate of the PIP joint.

Workup

Lateral plain radiographs are needed. If the dorsal portion of the articular surface of the middle phalanx is displaced dorsally on the head of the proximal phalanx, or if the joint pivots on the volar aspect of the intact remaining articular surface without sliding into flexion (revealing the V sign seen in the lateral plain radiograph), then an attempt at passive flexion to reduce the articular surfaces concentrically is indicated. A dorsal blocking splint with active and passive PIP flexion exercise is indicated, followed by gradual straightening of the dorsal block over the next 6 weeks. This is known as a *McElfresh technique* and can be used if joint reduction is concentric (the McElfresh technique should not be used if there is residual subluxation of the dorsal aspect of the middle phalanx).

Treatment

A McElfresh technique is attempted first. If reduction is unsuccessful, dynamic external fixation, internal fixation, volar plate arthroplasty, or hemihamate autograft arthroplasty can be performed. All result in some degree of fixed flexion deformity of the PIP joint.

Alternatives

In rare instances, the fracture may be left subluxated and allowed to remodel if the patient is pain free, if the fracture has not been diagnosed before union has occurred, and if motion is considered acceptable.

Principles and Clinical Pearls

- Early congruent articular reduction with early motion against a dorsal block or with a dynamic traction external fixator is optimal.
- Some degree of fixed flexion deformity is to be expected with any operative method for treatment of a subluxated joint.
- Sprained fingers should routinely be evaluated with a plain lateral radiograph early during the course of treatment.

Pitfalls

Pitfalls include persistent joint subluxation, osteoarthritis, frontal plane deformity, stiffness, weakness, pain, and tenderness.

Classic Reference

McElfresh EC, Dobyns JH, O'Brien ET. Management of fracture-dislocation of the proximal interphalangeal joints by extension-block splinting. J Bone Joint Surg Am 54:1705, 1972.
The McElfresh technique gained early and lasting acceptance for its simplicity and focus on obtaining and maintaining a concentric articular reduction without prolonged immobilization in PIP flexion.

48 Metacarpophalangeal Dislocation

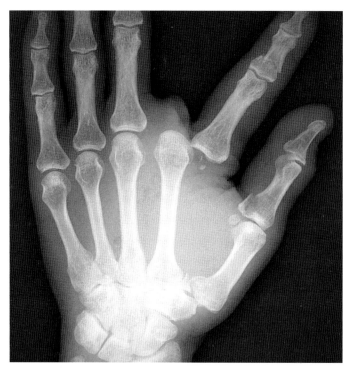

This 21-year-old collegiate rugby player was participating in a scrum when an opposing player forcibly hyperextended her index finger. She noted immediate pain and deformity in which the index finger was extended at the metacarpophalangeal (MCP) joint and deviated radially. She could not actively flex the finger at the MCP joint. She pulled on the finger almost immediately in an attempt to straighten it but was unsuccessful. On presentation to the emergency department, the patient had a prominence of the index metacarpal head in the distal radial aspect of her palm, and her proximal phalanx could not be reduced with appropriate anesthesia and traction on the finger. The volar skin puckered at the site of the dislocation. On a neurovascular examination, she had increased two-point discrimination on the radial aspect of her index finger pulp. An oblique radiograph is shown.

Description of the Problem

Irreducible MCP dislocations occur most often in either the index finger or the thumb. Although in rare occasions the base of the proximal phalanx can be volar to the head of the metacarpal, in most cases the injury is caused by hyperextension of the finger, and the base of the proximal phalanx rests dorsal to the head of the metacarpal.

Key Anatomy

The volar plate of the MCP joint is avulsed from its origin on the metacarpal neck and becomes interposed between the articular surface of the metacarpal head and the articular surface of the base of the proximal phalanx. The radial and ulnar collateral ligaments are rarely torn completely, and after reduction, the joint is usually mobile and stable.

Workup

PA, lateral, and oblique plain radiographs are obtained. If a transverse laceration is present over a dislocated MCP joint, then the joint is presumed to be open, and appropriate antibiotics and a tetanus prophylaxis are given. This usually consists of 2 g of cephalexin given intravenously and a tetanus toxoid given intramuscularly.

Treatment

Closed reduction is not possible if the volar plate is interposed, as described previously, and surgical reduction is required. If a dorsal approach is used, the interval between the index finger's extensor tendons (the extensor indicis proprius and the extensor digitorum communis) is approached, and the tendons are retracted ulnarly and radially, respectively. The dorsal capsule is usually stripped off of the metacarpal head and can be divided longitudinally or transversely. The head of the metacarpal is covered by an adherent volar plate, which has substantially less sheen than the articular cartilage. The volar plate is divided longitudinally using a scalpel and is then pushed back volarly using the dull end of the Freer elevator or an appropriately curved Farabeuf elevator. After the volar plate is reduced, the joint reduces easily. Skin and subcutaneous tissue are then closed and early active motion therapy initiated.

Alternatives

Open reduction using a volar approach is an alternative technique. The radial neurovascular bundle is tented over the metacarpal head and can be transected if the skin incision is too deep. The volar plate is identified at its insertion into the volar base of the proximal phalanx and delivered by traction into the wound. No repair is performed. The joint reduces easily, and skin and subcutaneous tissue are then closed. Postoperative care is identical to that of the dorsal approach described previously.

Principles and Clinical Pearls

- Longitudinal traction applied in the emergency department will not reduce the volar plate. Surgical exploration and direct operative reduction are needed.
- The volar approach places the radial digital nerve to the index finger at risk. Added care during the initial incision of the skin and subcutaneous tissue is appropriate.
- The dorsal approach and division of the dorsal capsule expose the metacarpal head. A hasty initial assessment may fool surgeons into believing they are looking at the metacarpal head, whose articular sheen has been dulled by the traumatic event. They are actually looking at the undersurface of the volar plate, which has been draped over the metacarpal head.

Pitfalls

A volar approach directly into the area where the radial nerve is tented over the metacarpal head and under the skin places the nerve at risk. A better alternative is to extend the approach proximally or distally in tissue where the nerve's position is not distorted and then trace the nerve into the field of injury.

Classic Reference

Bohart PG, Gelberman RH, Vandell RF, Salamon PB. Complex dislocations of the metacarpophalangeal joint. Clin Orthop Relat Res 164:208, 1982.
The authors conducted a retrospective analysis of nine complex MCP dislocations of the thumb and index finger performed through a dorsal approach. The volar plate was interposed between the head of the metacarpal and the base of the proximal phalanx in all cases; after reduction of the volar plate, a stable mobile joint reduction was achieved in all cases.

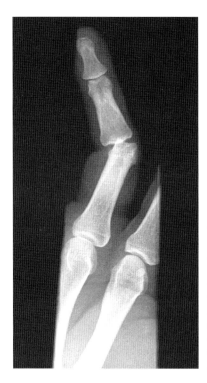

This 51-year-old surgeon injured the ring finger of his nondominant hand while playing third base in a recreational softball league. While attempting to stop a hard line drive, the glove was knocked off of his hand. He had immediate pain in the proximal interphalangeal (PIP) joint of his ring finger and noticed that the finger was hyperextended at this joint and deviated ulnarly. He pulled on the finger almost immediately in an attempt to straighten it but was unable to do so. On presentation to the emergency department, he had a prominence of the head of the proximal phalanx on the radial volar aspect of the finger, and it could not be reduced with a digital anesthesia block and direct traction on the finger. A neurovascular examination demonstrated normal sensation and capillary refill of the pulp and nail bed. An oblique radiograph is shown.

Description of the Problem

Irreducible (complex or rotatory) PIP dislocations occur as a result of a hyperextension and rotation force applied to the tip of the finger. Because of soft tissue interposed between the head of the proximal phalanx and the base of the middle phalanx, operative reduction is needed.

Key Anatomy

The volar plate is avulsed from the base of the middle phalanx, and one of the collateral ligaments is torn completely. The condyle of the head of the proximal phalanx is trapped between the lateral band and the central slip. Traction on the finger tightens the soft tissues around the head of the proximal phalanx and is ineffective in achieving reduction. Reduction requires the lateral band to be mechanically disengaged from between the proximal and middle phalanges.

Workup

PA, lateral, and oblique plain radiographs are obtained. A transverse laceration over the volar aspect of a dislocated PIP joint implies the joint is open, and appropriate antibiotics and a tetanus prophylaxis are given. This usually consists of 2 g of cephalexin given intravenously and a tetanus toxoid given intramuscularly.

Treatment

Closed reduction is not possible if the lateral band is interposed, as described previously, and surgical reduction is required. A dorsal approach is used, and the head of the proximal phalanx is identified subcutaneously. The central slip is identified inserting into the dorsal base of the middle phalanx and is preserved. The lateral band is identified proximally and traced into the zone of injury. It is then pulled dorsally (unhooking it from around the proximal phalangeal condyle) using a skin hook or a small elevator such as a Kleinert-Kutz elevator. After the lateral band is reduced, the joint reduces easily and is stable, if no associated articular fracture is identified. Skin and subcutaneous tissue are then closed and early active motion therapy initiated. On occasion, the PIP joint is immobilized in full extension for a short time to allow swelling to decrease and to prevent a fixed flexion deformity of the joint (a pseudo-boutonnière deformity).

Alternatives

Although operative open reduction of irreducible complex PIP dislocations is always needed, simple dislocations can be reduced easily and benefit from early motion therapy. An examination for integrity of the central slip and the triangular ligament after reduction helps to determine the need for splinting of the PIP joint. The ability to maintain a passively extended PIP joint in full active extension indicates whether the central slip and the triangular ligament are intact and whether immobilization in PIP extension (with or without a transarticular pin) is needed.

Principles and Clinical Pearls

- Longitudinal traction applied in the emergency department will not reduce a PIP joint. Surgical exploration and direct operative reduction are needed.
- A midaxial approach allows access to volar and dorsal structures.
- More commonly, dislocation of the base of the middle phalanx dorsally is accompanied by a fracture of the base of the middle phalanx volarly. If a substantial amount of the articular surface is fractured and displaced (generally between 30% and 50% of the articular surface), then the PIP joint reduction becomes difficult to obtain or maintain. Multiple methods of obtaining and maintaining reduction are available, including dorsal block splinting, dorsal block fixation, open reduction and internal fixation, hemihamate arthroplasty, volar plate arthroplasty, and dynamic traction.
- Hyperextension injuries of the PIP joint can result in soft tissue injuries without fractures. The integrity of the central slip and the triangular ligament can be assessed by the Elson Test, in which the PIP joint is flexed passively to 90 degrees, and active distal interphalangeal

Principles and Clinical Pearls—cont'd

joint extension is attempted. If the distal interphalangeal joint can be extended actively, the central slip and triangular ligament are NOT intact, and PIP extension splinting is needed. Another way to assess these structures is by placing the PIP joint passively into full extension and assessing the patient's ability to actively maintain the extended posture. If the patient is unable to do so, the central slip and triangular ligaments are disrupted, and a period of immobilization is needed after an open repair.

Pitfalls

Dorsal fracture dislocations of the PIP joint are common. Stable reduction of the joint is confirmed by an orthogonal lateral radiograph that demonstrates congruent articular surfaces. A dorsal V sign indicates incomplete reduction of the joint and the need for additional measures.

Classic Reference

Neviaser RJ, Wilson JN. Interposition of the extensor tendon resulting in persistent subluxation of the proximal interphalangeal joint of the finger. Clin Orthop Relat Res 83:118, 1972.
Irreducible PIP dislocations are discussed. Although rare, the extrication of the lateral band from the joint surgically is essential.

50 Scaphoid Fracture

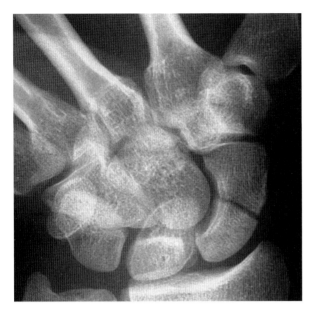

This 31-year-old bicyclist hit a pothole while traveling 5 miles per hour and was thrown over the front of his handlebars. He landed on his outstretched hand and felt pain immediately on the radial aspect of his wrist. He is otherwise well and has no history of wrist injury. He has a full-thickness skin abrasion over the base of his thenar eminence volarly and tenderness in the proximal aspect of the anatomic snuffbox. A comparison with the contralateral wrist reveals swelling in the anatomic snuffbox. A PA radiograph in ulnar deviation is shown. (Photo courtesy of Richard Gelberman, MD.)

Description of the Problem

The most common cause of fractures of the waist of the scaphoid is a fall onto an outstretched hand. High-energy dorsiflexion force applied to the radial wrist causes force transmission across the proximal carpal row, fracturing the scaphoid most frequently in a transverse pattern through the waist. This can result in distal pole fractures (rarely requiring operative treatment) and proximal pole fractures (which require operative fixation because of their tendency to result in nonunions if not surgically fixed). Fractures usually are not appreciated initially, and immobilization is delayed.

Key Anatomy

The radioscaphocapitate ligament crosses the waist of the scaphoid on its volar aspect and can serve as a fulcrum across which the scaphoid has a flexion moment applied and fails in tension. With a displaced scaphoid waist fracture, the intrascaphoid angle increases to more than its average of 45 degrees. The lunotriquetral ligament can be concurrently injured, resulting in an injury pattern known as a *transscaphoid perilunate fracture dislocation*. Infrequently, the scapholunate ligament is disrupted in a transscaphoid perilunate fracture dislocation. Although the scapholunate ligament is often intact with a scaphoid fracture, occasionally, the proximal scaphoid pole is devoid of bony or ligamentous attachment. This causes avascular necrosis of the proximal pole, which may affect bony and ligamentous healing adversely. The blood supply of the scaphoid originates primarily from the radial artery along its dorsal ridge and travels in a distal to proximal direction. The proximal pole supply is from the scapholunate ligament and the ligament of Testut (the radioscapholunate intracapsular ligament).

Workup

PA, lateral, and oblique plain radiographs are obtained. If a fracture is suspected but not visible radiographically, an MRI can be done. If surgical treatment of a nonunion is planned, a CT scan can be useful to assess the bone stock, the size of the fragments, and the degree of deformity and to determine the need for a bone graft.

Treatment

Open reduction and internal fixation of all proximal pole fractures should be performed; cast immobilization for distal pole fractures is sufficient. There is debate regarding fixation of nondisplaced waist fractures. Open reduction can be performed through a dorsal or a volar approach, arthroscopically (with a camera in the mid-carpal joint), or percutaneously. Headless screws are used. Once clinical and radiographic union is confirmed (as evidenced by bony bridging on a CT scan), wrist mobility and grip strength is addressed by synergistic grip–range of motion therapy and intermittent splinting. Passive stretching of the wrist to regain motion is not recommended.

Alternatives

If cast immobilization is undertaken, bony healing of nondisplaced scaphoid waist fractures can be expected by 8 to 14 weeks. The elbow and forearm can be immobilized, although no evidence proves its superiority over short-arm or thumb spica short-arm casting.

Principles and Clinical Pearls

- An early diagnosis will lead to earlier immobilization and probably an earlier union, compared with a late diagnosis.
- Either a dorsal or a volar approach can be performed, although a dorsal approach is preferred if the proximal pole is small or if a concurrent intercarpal ligament tear is treated. A volar approach is preferred if comminution is present at the waist and a volar bone graft is used.
- A scaphoid is not healed until it is healed radiographically; the best way to confirm this is with a CT scan through the longitudinal axis of the scaphoid.

Pitfalls

A late diagnosis, insufficient time of immobilization, and development of a nonunion can lead to adverse outcomes.

Classic Reference

Dias JJ, Wildin CJ, Bhowal B, Thompson JR. Should acute scaphoid fractures be fixed? A randomized controlled trial. J Bone Joint Surg Am 87:2160, 2005.
This compelling prospective randomized clinical trial discussed the benefits and risks of operative and nonoperative treatment of acute fractures of the waist of the scaphoid.

51 Scaphoid Nonunion

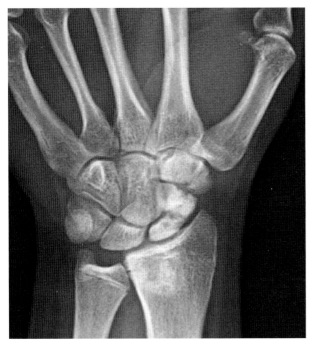

This 18-year-old college freshman slipped and fell at a campus party. She has wrist pain and swelling. She recalls that 2 years previously she injured her wrist while playing field hockey. At that time, a plain radiograph was obtained because of persistent pain. The film was interpreted as negative at the time, and her wrist was immobilized for 3 weeks. On examination, she has tenderness on palpation of her radioscaphoid joint and at the anatomic snuffbox. She has swelling over the dorsal aspect of her radiocarpal joint. Her wrist range of motion is painful in all planes but is decreased in extension and in radial deviation, compared with the contralateral side. A PA radiograph of the wrist is shown.

Description of the Problem

Nonunion of the waist of the scaphoid causes the proximal carpal row to become dissociated and allows the proximal pole of the scaphoid (along with the lunate) to become extended. On plain radiographs, this pattern of deformity is a dorsal intercalated segment instability, with the lunate extended (the radiolunate angle is increased in extension) and the capitolunate angle increased. Over time, arthritic changes develop, first within the radial styloid and the distal pole of the scaphoid and then within the scaphoid fossa of the distal radius. The capitolunate joint is affected next. The radiolunate joint is spared. This condition occurs after a missed diagnosis of a scaphoid waist fracture, followed by insufficient immobilization. The frequency with which the arthritic change becomes clinically relevant and symptomatic is unknown; however, it is generally accepted that if left undiagnosed, the arthritis will progress.

Key Anatomy

The scaphoid serves as a biomechanical link between the proximal and the distal carpal rows. A fracture of the scaphoid waist uncouples the proximal and the distal rows from one another and allows the lunate, which remains attached to the proximal pole of the scaphoid, to extend (dorsiflex). Extrinsic volar and dorsal ligamentous attachments to the lunate are insufficient to prevent lunate dorsiflexion, which occurs only because of the osseous anatomy of the carpus.

Workup

PA, lateral, ulnar deviation, and supinated clenched fist views of the wrist will show a scaphoid nonunion at various angles. A CT scan along the long axis of the scaphoid can be obtained for preoperative planning. If avascular necrosis of the proximal pole of the scaphoid is suspected, an MRI can be obtained if vascularized bone grafting is considered.

Treatment

Initial, nonoperative treatment for patients with a documented nonunion involves activity modification, a forearm-based splint (either custom-molded or off-the-shelf), and oral antiinflammatory agents given on a scheduled basis. Injections can be given for short-term control. Operative treatment is planned for patients whose symptoms are unrelieved by nonoperative means. Options include an open reduction, along with internal fixation and bone grafting for the scaphoid to restore scaphoid length and carpal anatomy and alignment; a scaphoid excision, as part of a proximal-row carpectomy or a capitate, lunate, hamate, and triquetrum (CLHT) fusion; and a total wrist arthrodesis or wrist arthroplasty.

Alternatives

Excision of the distal pole of the scaphoid can be combined with a radial styloidectomy if no capitolunate arthritis is noted on CT. A posterior interosseous neurectomy may decrease pain at the wrist joint.

Principles and Clinical Pearls

- A small proximal pole can be a surgical challenge. Although volar scaphoid bone grafting can be done, placing a screw retrograde into a small proximal pole is technically difficult.
- A vascularized dorsal distal radius graft can be useful if the proximal pole of the scaphoid is avascular.
- Some advocate temporary pinning of the radiolunate and/or the scaphocapitate joint during the postoperative period of immobilization.

Pitfalls

Scaphoid nonunion can occur even after bone grafting and open reduction and internal fixation. If a retrograde screw is placed through a starting point in the scaphotrapezial joint, then local arthritic changes can occur in this joint.

Classic Reference

Eggli S, Fernandez DL, Beck T. Unstable scaphoid fracture nonunion: a medium-term study of anterior wedge grafting procedures. J Hand Surg Br 27:36, 2002.

Although clinical and radiographic union was achieved in most patients, preexisting osteoarthritis was a predictor of poor results after correction of the nonunion.

52 Gunshot Wound to the Hand

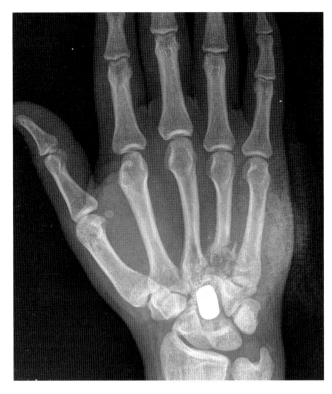

This patient has a small-caliber gunshot wound to the right hand and is seen in the emergency department. A PA radiograph of the hand and wrist is shown. (Photo courtesy of Jeff Yao, MD.)

Description of the Problem

In ballistic injuries to the hand, the amount of injury is dependent on the range, the caliber of the weapon, and the location of the bullet wound. The damage can involve multiple structures over a wide area. Understanding the mechanism of the injury and the resultant amount of trauma is critical for reconstructive purposes.

Key Anatomy

The bullet has entered the midcarpal region. The carpus and the base of the ring finger metacarpal are disrupted. In this region, the median and ulnar nerves and the flexor and extensor tendons may be damaged.

Workup

In patients with penetrating gunshot wounds to the hand, radiographs should be obtained to assess for the presence of an intact bullet. In many cases, the bullet has entered and exited the hand. A neurovascular examination is undertaken. Radiographs are also helpful for evaluating the bony injury. In most cases, emergent exploration is necessary to assess the damaged area.

Treatment

Based on this radiograph, the ring finger metacarpal bone is fractured and requires fixation. The bullet is present in the carpus. The entry and exit wounds should be explored by debriding necrotic tissue and excising proximally and distally, starting in normal tissue. Along the dorsal side, the extensor tendons should be assessed. Bony fractures should be explored. On the volar side, a carpal tunnel excision is made to assess the branches of the median nerve. Depending on the zone of injury, the ulnar nerve may also need to be explored. Flexor tendons are identified, and bony deficits are noted. K-wire fixation of the carpus may be a good initial maneuver given the comminution. Similarly, the metacarpal base can undergo K-wire fixation. If the hand is tense or if a large zone of injury is present, then hand fasciotomies are performed from a dorsal approach, ensuring that all intrinsic muscle compartments are released.

Failure to account for possible compartment syndrome may lead to a stiff and functionless hand (see Chapters 20 and 21). If a large amount of skin is necrotic, debridement may be necessary, and flap coverage should be performed soon thereafter.

Alternatives

In patients with through-and-through gunshot wounds in which the bullet has already exited, a careful physical examination is essential, noting all of the deficits. If no deficits are identified, then at times the hand may be observed. Primary nerve grafting is usually not recommended, because it is difficult to account for the zone of injury in these blast injuries.

Principles and Clinical Pearls

- In any gunshot wound, the range, the caliber, and the location should be noted.
- Identification of compartment syndromes is critical.
- In blast injuries, it is important to explore early; however, definitive reconstruction may need to be delayed until the zone of injury is determined.

Pitfalls

Compartment syndrome must be considered in cases of blast injuries to the hand. Failure to perform fasciotomies can lead to muscle necrosis. Early nerve grafting may result in poor nerve regeneration if the graft is placed across ends that are still damaged.

Classic References

Fackler ML, Burkhalter WE. Hand and forearm injuries from penetrating projectiles. J Hand Surg Am 17:971, 1992.
This was a classic review of hand and forearm penetrating injuries. The author provided an excellent discussion of the wound profiles caused by different caliber bullets.

Langford M, Cheung K, Li Z. Percutaneous distraction pinning for metacarpophalangeal joint stabilization after blast or crush injuries of the hand. Clin Orthop Relat Res 473:2785.
The metacarpophalangeal joint may be destroyed in cases of blast injuries because of the location in the center of the hand. The authors discussed external fixation devices to hold the joint at length.

Turker T, Capdarest-Arest N. Management of gunshot wounds to the hand: a literature review. J Hand Surg Am 38:1641, 2013.
This was an excellent recent review of the management of gunshot wounds to the hand. The authors discussed the timing of treatment and indications for surgery.

53 Hook of Hamate Fracture

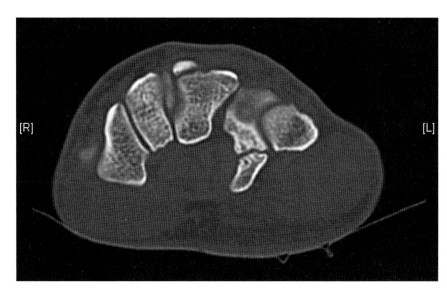

This CT image shows a 32-year-old man who hurt his right wrist while golfing 8 weeks ago. He has nonspecific aching. On examination, point tenderness is noted over the hook of the hamate. Plain radiographs are inconclusive. An axial view of the carpus is shown.

Description of the Problem

A fracture of the hook of the hamate is common in golfers who hit the turf; in baseball players, because of the shock of the batted ball; and in cyclists who fall onto their hands. There may be some aching in the area, but because there is no deformity or displacement, the injury may go untreated. As the aching pain persists, patients may seek care from general practitioners, who order radiographs. The radiographs are commonly read as *normal,* because the hook of the hamate is superimposed on the rest of the hamate. Patients present to a hand surgeon weeks to months after the injury. By this time, a nonunion has developed.

Key Anatomy

The hook of the hamate juts volarly from the main body of the hamate. It forms the radial border of the Guyon canal and is directly adjacent to the ulnar nerve and artery. The flexor tendons to the small finger course ulnarly around the radial aspect of this hook, which acts as a pivot point. Surgery to excise the hook of the hamate requires careful identification and preservation of the deep motor branch of the ulnar nerve. Because the base of the hook is narrow and motion occurs in the palm, immobilization until the fracture has healed is difficult.

Workup

Patients are referred to a hand surgeon. They typically have aching pain in the ulnar/volar wrist and tenderness resting the palm while using the computer, weight lifting, and with other daily activities. Tenderness is localized over the hook of the hamate with deep palpation. A carpal tunnel view on plain radiographs may show the fracture at the base of the hook. If a radiograph is not conclusive, CT or MRI will reveal the fracture.

Treatment

Patients with a recent injury may opt for a 4-week period of immobilization with a wrist cast. This is reasonable, because the definitive treatment may require removal of the hook of the hamate. If the immobilization is unsuccessful or if the presentation is late, then surgical excision of the hook of the hamate is recommended.

Surgery begins with a longitudinal incision over the hook of the hamate. Fluoroscopy may aid in correct placement of the incision over the hook. The ulnar nerve, especially the motor branch, is always identified. The tip of the hook is dissected, and subperiosteal dissection continues deeper until the nonunion is encountered. The ulnar nerve is constantly visualized and gently retracted. A Freer elevator is useful for teasing out the nonunion site, and the hook is gently removed in one piece. The remaining base is examined for sharp edges, which are rongeured. The surgeon should note that the hook of the hamate is larger than one would imagine.

After the excision is finished, the ulnar nerve is inspected to ensure it has not been injured. The small finger flexor tendons are examined for signs of rupture or damage from the fracture site.

Alternatives

A patient may not seek treatment if the wrist is nontender. This is acceptable, because no functional problem exists. Some surgeons have advocated reduction and fixation of the fracture. This is not recommended, because a hook of the hamate fracture is difficult to heal, and the ulnar nerve is placed at unnecessary risk. These patients usually do very well without the hook of the hamate.

Principles and Clinical Pearls

- This injury is difficult to detect on plain radiographs. Palpation of point tenderness and CT/MRI are most diagnostic.
- The ulnar nerve must be identified and protected at all times.
- Removal of the hook of the hamate requires deep dissection of a large portion of the bone.

Pitfalls

A fracture of the hook of the hamate can be incompletely excised if the surgeon does not appreciate the size of the bone. The most dreaded complication is damage to the motor branch of the ulnar nerve. Even if it is not directly cut, excessive retraction may cause temporary paralysis of the intrinsic muscles.

Classic References

Klausmeyer M, Mudgal C. Hook of hamate fractures. J Hand Surg 38:2457, 2013.
This recent review of the topic discussed imaging modalities and the arguments for open reduction and internal fixation versus excision of the fractured hook. The authors correctly commented that good evidence is difficult to obtain because of the late presentation and small numbers in each series.

Yamazaki H, Kato H, Nakatsuchi N, Murakami N, Hata Y. Closed rupture of the flexor tendons of the little finger secondary to non-union of fractures of the hook of the hamate. J Hand Surg Br 31:337, 2006.
In this paper, the authors compiled six cases of little finger flexor tendon rupture after nonunion of the hook of the hamate. The site of the nonunion included the tip (1), the midportion (3) and the base (2). Therefore tendon rupture can be caused by a nonunion anywhere along the hook. Secondary tendon reconstruction would be needed.

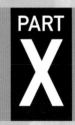

PART

X

Infections/Bites

54 Human Bite Injury

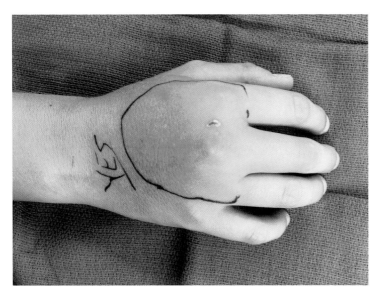

This 24-year-old student presents to the emergency department with a 36-hour history of pain, swelling, redness, and fever from a laceration to the dorsal aspect of the skin overlying the third metacarpophalangeal (MCP) joint of his right, dominant hand. Initially, the patient denies a history of trauma. His companion corrects him by recalling an altercation in which the patient struck an assailant with a closed fist after a night of heavy drinking at a local pub. The pain and swelling have increased gradually since that time. He is febrile at 39.6° C and has a 1 cm transverse laceration over the dorsum of his middle ray MCP joint. A small amount of pus is expressed from the laceration, and the dorsum of the hand is swollen, red, and tender. Lymphangitic streaks extend proximally up the dorsum of the forearm, and an epitrochlear node is palpated just proximal to the elbow on the medial side. He is unable to extend the finger actively.

Description of the Problem

Human bite injuries (so-called fight bites) occur over the dorsum of the hand at the level of the second, third, or fourth MCP joints. They result from striking a closed fist over the tooth of the assailant and the inoculation of polymicrobial oral flora in either the MCP joint or the surrounding soft tissue (or both). Occasionally, a fragment of broken tooth is lodged in the MCP joint cartilage or in the surrounding soft tissues.

Key Anatomy

The hand is in a position of MCP, proximal interphalangeal, and distal interphalangeal flexion (a closed fist) at the moment of impact, and the extensor mechanism (the extrinsic digital extensor tendon and the sagittal bands) is pulled distally. The laceration in the joint capsule may be obscured by the tendon retracting proximally as the fist is released.

Workup

PA, lateral, and oblique plain radiographs are obtained. Intraarticular gas and pieces of tooth are sought. A culture for aerobic and anaerobic organisms and a Gram stain are sent.

Treatment

Operative treatment requires wound excision and extensor tendon repair (if necessary) and joint exploration, debridement, and direct irrigation. Prolonged exposure and dessication of the articular cartilage should be avoided; however, the cutaneous wound should never be fully closed primarily after incision and drainage.

Alternatives

There is no alternative treatment to operative exploration, irrigation, and drainage of the MCP joint.

Principles and Clinical Pearls

- The history that a patient provides on presentation is often (purposefully) inaccurate.
- An untreated wound can result in septic arthritis with loss of articular cartilage, metacarpal head osteomyelitis, and a dorsal skin and soft tissue defect.
- Antibiotic treatment never takes precedence over surgical exploration, irrigation, and debridement.

Pitfalls

Pitfalls include inadequate exposure, irrigation, debridement, or drainage. Although local or other flap coverage might be required later, aggressive resection of infected, dead, and/or devitalized tissue is essential.

Classic Reference

Mennen U, Howells CJ. Human fight-bite injuries of the hand. A study of 100 cases within 18 months. J Hand Surg Br 16:431, 1991.

In a study of 100 consecutive cases, the authors reported an astonishing rate of 18% amputation. They stressed early, thorough, and repeated debridement of infected MCP joints.

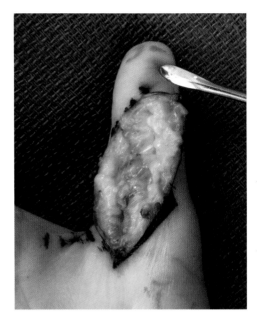

This 36-year-old executive recruiter presented to her primary care physician's office 10 hours after being bitten by the family cat. She had been holding the cat, when the animal became scared and bit her several times over the thenar eminence, the thumb metacarpophalangeal (MCP) joint, and the proximal phalanx of the thumb. Initially, the wounds appeared small and punctate; however, over the past 3 hours, they have become increasingly painful, red, and swollen. Motion of the MCP joint is extremely painful, and red streaks have appeared, extending proximally from the puncture site over the MCP joint. She has a low-grade fever and malaise.

Description of the Problem

Feline teeth are long and sharp, and a cat bite has been likened to a subdermal (intraarticular, intrasynovial, or intraosseous) inoculation of feline oral bacteria. The shape of feline teeth and the soft tissue damage caused by a cat bite are distinct from the damage caused by a dog bite, which tends to have a more broadly based entry wound and tearing in terms of mechanism. The most frequently isolated organism from cat-bite wounds is *Pasteurella multocida* (subspecies *septica* and *multocida*); however, polymicrobial cultures are frequently seen.

Key Anatomy

Feline teeth penetrate deeply and can penetrate the skin in nonorthogonal directions. Any entry wound near a joint or tendon sheath should be presumed to involve the closed space until determined otherwise.

Workup

PA, lateral, and oblique plain radiographs are obtained. If only skin or soft tissue inoculation is suspected, a sample for culture may be obtained under sterile conditions by unroofing the entry wound with a hypodermic 25-gauge or 27-gauge needle.

Treatment

An oral antibiotic such as Augmentin can be useful for prophylaxis, and a beta-lactam, combined with a beta-lactamase inhibitor, can be given intravenously. The patient's tetanus immunization status is updated. If an intraarticular or an intrasynovial infection is present, operative drainage and irrigation are needed, followed by intravenous antibiotics against the cultured organisms.

Alternatives

A bacterial culture should always be obtained, and antibiotic treatment should be directed toward the most populous organism. Whether to carry out surgical drainage depends on the surgeon's discretion; however, vigilance against deep infection should always be a priority because of the unique anatomy of feline teeth.

Principles and Clinical Pearls

- Feline teeth are long and sharp—they penetrate deeply into soft tissues and can penetrate the joint capsule.
- Although a sterile reactive arthritis can result from a cat bite in the vicinity of a joint, these wounds should be treated as if the joint has been penetrated and a bacterial septic arthritis is present.
- Patients with cat bites frequently have multiple entry wounds. Each wound should be examined for the presence of a deep infection or a closed-space infection.

Pitfalls

A delay in giving antibiotics or in surgical treatment can result in increased tissue damage.

Classic Reference

Talan DA, Citron DM, Abrahamian FM, Moran GJ, Goldstein EJ. Bacteriologic analysis of infected dog and cat bites. Emergency Medicine Animal Bite Infection Study Group. N Engl J Med 340:85, 1999.
The organism most frequently isolated from dog and cat bites was Pasteurella multocida, although multiple aerobic and anaerobic species were identified in both types of bite wound.

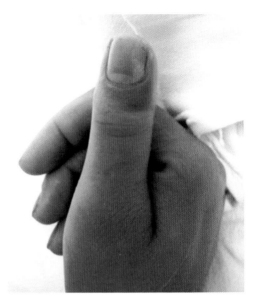

This 16-year-old nail biter presents to his pediatrician with a 3-day history of progressive pain, swelling, redness, and warmth along the radial aspect of the eponychial fold of his right dominant index finger. His mother had expressed a small amount of pus from the area of the inflammation. She explains that soaks in warm water with Epsom salts had provided him with little relief. He is afebrile and has no swelling or tenderness in the pulp of the finger or along the flexor tendon sheath.

Description of the Problem

A paronychia is a localized infection within the soft tissue space between the nail plate and the eponychial fold. It frequently begins as a localized inflammatory process but progresses to a collection of pus and can extend around the radial or ulnar aspect of the distal phalanx to cause a felon (pulp space abscess) to develop. In diabetic patients and those who are immunocompromised, paronychia can cause a flexor tendon sheath infection and a septic arthritis of the distal interphalangeal (DIP) joint.

Key Anatomy

A collection of pus in the soft tissue between the deep aspect of the eponychial fold overlying the proximal aspect of the nail plate (which overlies the germinal nail matrix) and between the superficial and deep aspects of the eponychial folds distinguishes a paronychia from a felon (a collection of pus within the volar pulp space of the finger), a flexor tendon sheath infection (a collection of pus between the visceral and parietal paratenon of the flexor sheath), and septic arthritis of the DIP joint (a collection of pus within the DIP joint, often associated with osteomyelitis of the distal phalanx).

Workup

PA, lateral, and oblique plain radiographs are obtained to check for osteomyelitis or bone resorption. If a sample of the pus can be obtained with little discomfort for the patient, then a swab is sent for culture and sensitivity testing and a Gram stain. In chronic cases, additional fungal cultures should be obtained.

Treatment

If an abscess is present, surgical drainage is performed under sterile conditions, with the patient anesthetized with a digital block. Additional samples are sent for culture and sensitivity testing, and broad-spectrum antibiotics are given either orally (if the infection is localized) or intravenously (if the infection has invaded bone, the joint, or the flexor sheath.) If an abscess is not present, an oral antibiotic can be given.

Alternatives

If an abscess requires drainage, an oblique incision is carried proximally, extending from the proximoradial or the proximoulnar aspect of the eponychium into the abscess cavity. This allows direct drainage of the pus, and the wound can heal by secondary intention, ensuring continued drainage of purulent and necrotic material, if indicated. If a felon is also present, a midline longitudinal incision over the pulp space (between the terminal branches of the radial and the ulnar digital nerves) is advisable. If septic arthritis of the DIP joint is present, a direct approach to the DIP joint through the area of "pointing" of the associated abscess is recommended, rather than creating additional devascularized skin flaps and soft tissue planes.

Principles and Clinical Pearls

- Decompression with the patient under a local anesthetic given as a digital block, followed by oral antibiotic treatment, is often all that is needed.
- Undertreatment in the form of nonsurgical management carries greater risk than early surgical decompression and treatment with oral or intravenous antibiotics, especially in diabetic or immunocompromised patients.
- Chronic cases can be the result of a *Candida* or other fungal superinfection and might need to be treated by nail plate removal and eponychial marsupialization.

Pitfalls

Incomplete drainage or administration of antibiotics that were not verified by evaluation of culture and sensitivity testing may lead to continued infection.

Classic Reference

Shafritz AB, Coppage JM. Acute and chronic paronychia of the hand. J Am Acad Orthop Surg 22:165, 2014.
This useful current review article outlined surgical and antimicrobial treatment.

57 Herpetic Whitlow

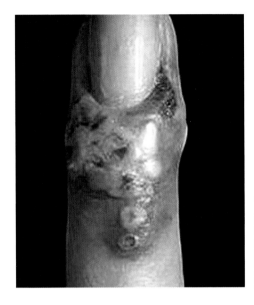

This 41-year-old respiratory therapist presents to her primary care physician with a 3-day history of a painful vesicular rash over the eponychium and pulp skin of her right dominant middle finger. She describes the pain as burning, and the skin surrounding the vesicles is red and intensely irritated. The content of the vesicles appears to be clear and colorless; however, she has not attempted to rupture the lesion, because it is too painful to touch.

Description of the Problem

Herpetic whitlow is a cutaneous infection caused by herpes simplex type 1 and less frequently by herpes simplex type 2. It is seen frequently in health care workers and is probably caused by a local inoculation from an exposure to fluid secretions containing the virus. Its appearance is characteristically a collection of small, clear, and thin-walled vesicles over a tender, erythematous base. No pus is present, and bacterial superinfection occurs only if vesicular rupture is attempted. The vesicular contents can become turbid or hemorrhagic but should not be mistaken for pus.

Key Anatomy

The infection is confined to the epidermis and dermis.

Workup

Serology for viral culture, polymerase chain reaction testing for viral nucleotide sequences, and immunofluorescence for herpes simplex virus antigen can be carried out. Frequently, the appearance is characteristic of herpes simplex viral infection, and further testing is not required.

Treatment

Without treatment, these lesions will heal in 2 to 3 weeks. Oral antiviral agents such as acyclovir or topical acyclovir may be given to immunocompromised patients. Treatment with acyclovir during the prodromal phase of symptoms can decrease the length of the attack and its severity.

Alternatives

There are no treatment alternatives. A bacterial infection should be ruled out based on the history and physical findings.

Principles and Clinical Pearls

- Diagnosis is most often made on the basis of a physical examination alone.
- An immunofluorescent evaluation of vesicle fluid with commercially available assays can confirm the diagnosis in questionable cases.

Pitfalls

Treatment with oral or topical antibiotics, assuming the infection is bacterial and responsive to antibacterial agents, is ill-advised. Aggressive incision and drainage of vesicles is both painful and valueless.

Classic Reference

Rubright JH, Shafritz AB. The herpetic whitlow. J Hand Surg Am 36:340, 2011.
The authors provided an excellent review of the pathologic causes, the diagnosis, and the treatment of whitlows.

58 Flexor Tenosynovitis

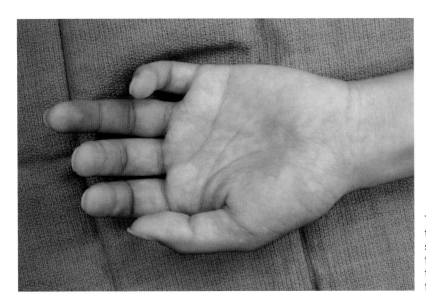

This 32-year-old man is seen in the emergency department with a slightly swollen and tender left ring finger. He had been gardening over the weekend and may have punctured his finger.

Description of the Problem

The patient has an extended and painful left ring finger. Suspicion of flexor tenosynovitis should be high. In this infection, the bacteria are trapped within the flexor tendon sheath. This causes pain and swelling along the course of the sheath.

Key Anatomy

The anatomy of the flexor tendon sheath determines the etiology of the problem. Penetrating bacteria can infiltrate the space between the sheath and flexor tendon. The infection is trapped inside this sheath, with no ability to be decompressed. As the infection develops, the swelling and pain will proceed proximally along the flexor tendon sheath into the palm and even more proximally into the wrist at Parona's space, which is the flexor tendon space directly above the pronator quadratus muscle.

Workup

PA, lateral, and oblique radiographs are obtained to assess for a foreign body. Patients are examined for the classic Kanavel's signs, which include (1) fusiform swelling of the digit, (2) pain with motion of the digits, (3) a semiflexed position, and (4) exquisite tenderness along the sheath.

Treatment

If purulent drainage from the digit is noted, then emergent operative treatment is needed. If no drainage is noted, treatment involves splint immobilization of the hand, elevation, and intravenous antibiotics. The patient is admitted for overnight observation and is taken to the operating room the next morning if the pain and swelling have not resolved. Surgery requires opening the flexor tendon sheath proximally and distally and irrigating the flexor tendon sheath with an antibiotic solution. A splint is placed in the position of safety (wrist extended 30 degrees, MCP joints flexed 90 degrees, and IP joints straight), and the patient is followed for the possibility of a second-look operation.

Alternatives

Alternative incisions can be made for a flexor tenosynovitis release. Although we advocate a small distal incision at the distal interphalangeal joint and another incision in the palm to irrigate the sheath, some surgeons prefer to perform a midlateral incision along the entire finger or Bruner's incisions in a zigzag fashion along the entire finger. Furthermore, some place a temporary irrigation catheter to allow flushing of the sheath.

Principles and Clinical Pearls

- Understanding the tight anatomy of the flexor tendon sheath will inform the surgeon of the pathophysiology.
- Patients can be observed overnight but should be operated on if the problem has not resolved by the morning.
- Resolution of this infection is essential to prevent stiffness in the future.

Pitfalls

Pitfalls are related to missing the diagnosis of flexor tenosynovitis. If the infection becomes severe, it can spread around the bursa to the entire hand and into the forearm. When making the incisions, care is critical to prevent damage to the digital arteries and nerve and to the flexor tendons.

Classic References

Giladi AM, Malay S, Chung KC. A systematic review of the management of acute pyogenic flexor tenosynovitis. J Hand Surg Eur Vol 40:720, 2015.
The authors conducted a systematic review of the management of flexor tenosynovitis. The studies showed the benefit of early treatment of pyogenic flexor tenosynovitis and systemic antibiotic use.

Jing SS, Iyer S. Simplifying irrigation in flexor tenosynovitis. J Hand Surg Eur Vol 40:321, 2015.
The authors described a simple technique for irrigating flexor tenosynovitis using an ear suction catheter. Cannulas seemed ideal for this indication.

Lille S, Hayakawa T, Neumeister MW, Brown RE, Zook EG, Murray K. Continuous postoperative catheter irrigation is not necessary for the treatment of suppurative flexor tenosynovitis. J Hand Surg Br 25:304, 2000.
The authors reviewed their series of patients with pyogenic flexor tenosynovitis and found that continuous postoperative irrigation was not necessary.

59 Osteomyelitis

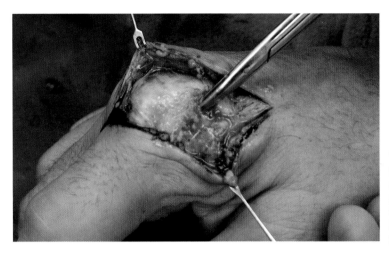

This man is seen intraoperatively with purulent drainage from the metacarpal head of his index finger. He received a nail gun puncture injury to his hand 1 week ago and has had increasing pain and swelling around the index finger metacarpophalangeal (MCP) joint.

Description of the Problem

The patient has acute osteomyelitis of the metacarpal head. He has destruction of the bone from a bacterial infection.

Key Anatomy

The MCP joint is critical for range of motion for the hand. This patient developed osteomyelitis of the metacarpal head and destruction of the cartilage surface of the MCP joint. This will lead to progressive collapse of the joint and poor range of motion of the index finger.

Workup

PA, lateral, and oblique radiographs are required. They may reveal lucency in the bone related to bacteria. The hand is examined for swelling, redness, and pain. Pain with range of motion may implicate involvement of the joint.

The presence of a draining wound necessitates emergent surgery for drainage and debridement. Routine cultures are sent. The history is a critical part of the workup. Patients should be asked about recent travel, their occupation, activities, and comorbid medical conditions. A fight-bite injury may have inoculated bacteria into the joint (see Chapter 54).

Treatment

A deep infection of the hand is suspected in this patient; therefore he needs emergent incision and drainage to preserve the joint surfaces and to prevent osteomyelitis. Surgery should begin with an incision in the area and extension of the incision proximally and distally to normal tissue planes. Specifically around the MCP joint, the extensor tendon is dissected and lifted to assess for infection. The sagittal band may need to be partially released to access the region.

If joint infection is suspected, the joint is opened. In this case, radiographs showed lucency of the metacarpal head; therefore coring of the metacarpal head was performed to promote drainage of the bacteria. The patient underwent copious irrigation with an antibiotic solution, and the wound was partially closed. Significant bone destruction that requires removal of a portion of the metacarpal head can benefit from the placement of an antibiotic spacer, which maintains the joint area while helping to rid the region of infection.

Alternatives

There is no treatment alternative to operative debridement for osteomyelitis. Debridement of all necrotic and infected bone is critical.

Principles and Clinical Pearls

- A fight-bite injury or other puncture wound may inoculate human mouth flora underneath the extensor tendon and into the joint or into the region around the metacarpal head. A carefully obtained history of a recent fight and early antibiotic treatment with debridement, as indicated, are essential to prevent joint infection and/or osteomyelitis.
- In patients with osteomyelitis, necrotic bone must be removed, although this can lead to a very difficult reconstruction.
- The MCP joint is critical for range of motion of the hand toward making a fist.

Pitfalls

Pitfalls are related to poor vigilance regarding the possibility of joint infection or osteomyelitis. Once an infection attacks the cartilage surface and the bone, reconstruction of a normal bone and joint is difficult.

Classic References

Kowalski TJ, Thompson LA, Gundrum JD. Antimicrobial management of septic arthritis of the hand and wrist. Infection 42:379, 2014.
This was an excellent review from the infectious disease literature on proper antimicrobial treatment for joint infections of the hand and wrist.

Micev A, Kalainov DM, Soneru AP. Masquelet technique for treatment of segmental bone loss in the upper extremity. J Hand Surg Am 40:593, 2015.
Micev and his coauthors reviewed the Masquelet technique for treating segmental bone loss in the hand and upper extremity. In this technique, the fibrous membrane that forms after placement of a cement spacer is preserved and used to hold cancellous bone graft in the second stage.

Okada M, Kamano M, Uemura T, Ikeda M, Nakamura H. Pedicled adipose tissue for treatment of chronic digital osteomyelitis. J Hand Surg Am 40:677, 2015.
Digital osteomyelitis can lead to wound coverage issues because of the extensive debridement that may be necessary. The authors presented a technique of coverage for this digital osteomyelitis using a pedicled adipose tissue flap.

60 Necrotizing Fasciitis

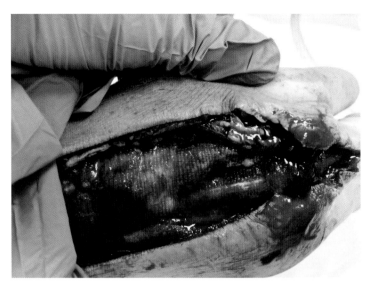

This 28-year-old woman presents to the emergency department 2 days after closing a closet door on the dorsum of her left, nondominant hand. She noticed a small abrasion where the door had struck her hand, but thought nothing of it at the time. Over the next 24 hours, she noted increased swelling, pain, and crepitus over the abrasion. She also had a low-grade fever. The next night, she felt increasingly unwell systemically, and noticed further swelling, pain, redness, and severe tenderness over the area of the abrasion and extending proximally across her wrist. Her temperature was elevated to 39.7° F. The following morning, she presents to the emergency department. On examination, her blood pressure is 85/50 mm Hg, her pulse is 140 beats/min and regular, and her respiratory rate is 40 breaths/min. She is alert and oriented and appears acutely ill. Her arm is grossly swollen. She cannot move her fingers and has altered sensation in her fingers. A small amount of serosanguinous discharge is draining from the dorsal abrasion. The dorsum of the hand is incised and widely opened.

Description of the Problem

A rapidly progressive infection of the hand and arm that develops after a seemingly inconsequential injury to the skin is typical of a necrotizing infection involving the fascia and the skin. Deeper tissues such as muscle and intracompartmental structures are involved less frequently in the absence of an open fracture. The most commonly involved infectious agents are *Staphylococcus* and *Streptococcus*.

Key Anatomy

The infection spreads along the fascial planes deep to the skin and the dermis.

Workup

Hemodynamic stabilization is the first priority for patients with necrotizing fasciitis. Fluids and pressor agents are given as necessary during the workup. PA, lateral, and oblique plain radiographs are obtained. Swelling and gas in the soft tissues are sought. An emergent Gram stain is sent to evaluate for gram-positive organisms or anaerobic organisms, and fluid is sent for culture. Patients should be prepped for the operating room as quickly as possible, because rapid drainage, debridement, and irrigation are the mainstays of treatment of this potentially fatal infection.

Treatment

After the vital signs have stabilized, a surgical incision is made on the involved extremity. The initial traumatic wound is excised. The incision is extended through skin, subcutaneous tissues, and fascia to the level of normal tissue throughout the infected area up the hand, wrist, forearm, and arm. The wounds are irrigated thoroughly and left open. Intravenous antibiotics are given, first broad-spectrum and then based on the specificity and sensitivity data of microbial isolates. Closure or split-thickness skin grafting is not attempted until the infection is controlled, and the patient's hemodynamic status has normalized. Occasionally, the infection is so severe that the only way to stop the progression is by amputation of the affected extremity.

Alternatives

There is no treatment alternative to surgical debridement, drainage, irrigation, and intravenous antibiotics. Rarely, hyperbaric oxygen treatment is an option for a severe anaerobic infection.

Principles and Clinical Pearls

- Early diagnosis and surgical treatment are critical to prevent long-term disability, amputation, and death.
- Beta-hemolytic streptococcus, *S. aureus,* and mixed, polymicrobial infections are most common.
- Aggressive surgical treatment is required. Surgeons should never rely on antibiotics to do what they have not been able to do surgically.
- Frequent trips to the operating room may be necessary to control and eradicate the infection. There is no "right" number of surgeries needed to control infection and prevent limb loss.

Pitfalls

Too-minimal surgical debridement can allow the infection to spread rapidly, thus endangering limb and life. Incorrect antibiotic administration based on sensitivity and specificity data can cost the surgeon valuable time needed for bacterial eradication. Antibiotics can only penetrate tissues that are perfused. They do not kill bacteria in necrotic or hypoperfused tissue.

Classic Reference

Gonzalez MH, Kay T, Weinzweig N, Brown A, Pulvirenti J. Necrotizing fasciitis of the upper extremity. J Hand Surg Am 21:689, 1996.
An early report in the hand surgical literature discussed the severe nature of this condition, its potential to spread rapidly, and the possible need for forequarter amputation.

61 Chronic Olecranon Bursitis

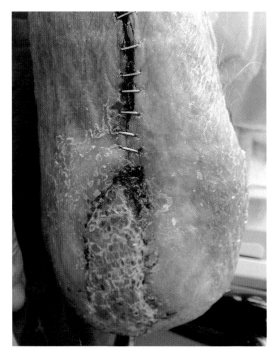

This 70-year-old man presents to the office with a mass over his posterior elbow. It is painful and swollen and has been draining for 3 weeks. He had presented to his primary care physician 3 weeks ago with a swollen mass over the olecranon, with no history of trauma or discomfort. The physician elected to drain the fluid from the mass with the patient under a local anesthetic. Twenty milliliters of yellow, blood-tinged synovial fluid was drained. Since that time, the patient has developed increasing pain, loss of elbow range of motion in flexion (from pain and tightness posteriorly), and a low-grade fever and malaise. Cloudy, serosanguinous fluid was drained from a 2.5 cm wound directly over the posterior aspect of the olecranon. A total bursectomy and a flexor carpi ulnaris flap and split-thickness skin graft were performed, as shown.

Description of the Problem

Chronic olecranon bursitis is a benign condition and should, in most cases, be managed by nonoperative methods such as an elbow pad. Interventions such as needle or incisional drainage frequently lead to chronic leakage of synovial fluid or nonhealing wounds that require more aggressive surgical treatment.

Key Anatomy

The olecranon bursa overlies the triceps tendon insertion and the olecranon directly. Typically, the skin over the posterior elbow is subjected to repeated trauma and can develop small cracks through which bacteria can inoculate the bursa and subcutaneous tissue directly. This is infrequent, however, and most cases of olecranon bursitis are sterile and nonpainful. Intraarticular involvement of the elbow joint is a concern only in patients with rheumatoid arthritis or gout. In such cases, triceps tendon involvement is common, and more extensive joint and soft tissue debridement and irrigation are needed.

Workup

PA, lateral, and oblique plain radiographs are obtained. The presence of gas in the soft tissues and joint space narrowing of the ulnohumeral or radiocapitellar joint are sought. Fluid draining on presentation should be sent for microbiologic analysis. Rarely, the cause is a mycobacterial or fungal infection or crystal deposition, and microbiologic and histologic evaluations are required.

Treatment

Treatment involves resection of the entire olecranon bursa, followed by soft tissue closure or flap coverage of the skin defect. Postoperatively, the elbow should be immobilized in full extension or nearly full extension until the longitudinal incision over the posterior elbow has completely healed. If flap closure is necessary, several reliable choices are available: an anconeus muscle, a flexor carpi ulnaris muscle, or a radial forearm fasciocutaneous flap. The photograph shows the coverage that can be expected with a flexor carpi ulnaris flap covered by a split-thickness skin graft.

Alternatives

Noninterventional treatment of chronic olecranon bursitis is preferred unless the wound is infected. Occasionally, a mass is large enough to cause difficulty with clothing or other mass-effect considerations. For these patients, needle drainage is performed under sterile conditions, followed by strict compression and elbow immobilization in extension.

Principles and Clinical Pearls

- If a decision to excise the bursa is made, a total bursectomy through a wide extensile surgical approach is necessary.
- Nonoperative treatment with antiinflammatories, compression, and immobilization is preferred for initial presentations.
- Too-early or injudicious mobilization of the elbow after a posterior incision can result in wound dehiscence and the development of a chronic soft tissue wound.

Pitfalls

Surgeons should resist the urge toward interventional and/or surgical treatment of this condition unless an infection that needs to be surgically drained or a chronic draining wound is present.

Classic Reference

Sayegh ET, Strauch RJ. Treatment of olecranon bursitis: a systematic review. Arch Orthop Trauma Surg 134:1517, 2014.

Based on mostly Level IV evidence, the authors advocated nonoperative treatment as being more effective than operative treatment for patients with chronic sterile olecranon bursitis.

Infections/Extravasations

62 Dorsal Hand Extravasation

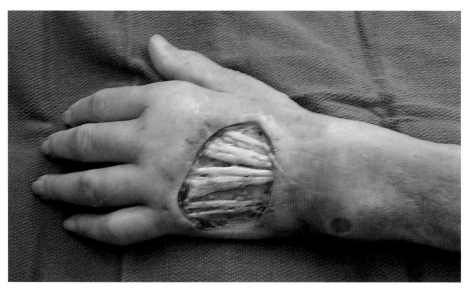

This patient has undergone debridement after an intravenous extravasation of chemotherapeutic agents into the dorsal hand.

Description of the Problem

The patient has a full-thickness dorsal hand wound. The dorsal hand skin is susceptible to intravenous extravasation injuries. The extensor tendons are intact but desiccated and require coverage.

Key Anatomy

The dorsal skin is very thin and pliable, which allows gliding of the extensor tendons. It is susceptible to avulsion injuries and extravasation injuries. The extensor tendons are freely gliding distal to the extensor retinaculum. They are connected by juncturae tendinum, which promote synchronous motion. The paratenon to the extensor tendons is very thin. Once it is destroyed, exposure will lead to extensor tendon desiccation and rupture. Furthermore, scarring of the extensor tendons will prevent adequate flexion at the metacarpophalangeal joints. Secondary metacarpophalangeal joint scarring can occur, contributing to stiffness in extension of the joint.

Workup

The patient requires a careful wound evaluation for evidence of infection or purulent drainage. The paratenon is evaluated. If the tendons are intact but the paratenon is missing, then the patient will need flap coverage. Skin grafting will not be adequate. Several flaps are available, based on the radial artery. Therefore an Allen test should be performed to assess the patency of the arch and the communication between the ulnar and radial arteries. The volar forearm skin is evaluated.

Treatment

Dorsal hand coverage is categorized according to the requirements on the dorsum. If only the skin is involved and the extensor tendons are intact, then a radial forearm fascia-only flap is preferred. This will allow transfer of the radial forearm fascia in a retrograde fashion based on the radial artery. The fascia can be transferred to the dorsal side and covered with a split-thickness, unmeshed skin graft. This re-creates the dorsal skin with minimal bulk. However, if the dorsal hand has lost the extensor tendons, then thicker tissue needs to be placed to allow future secondary procedures such as extensor tendon grafting. In this case, a traditional reverse radial forearm fasciocutaneous flap is the treatment of choice.

Alternatives

Alternatives to the radial forearm options are available. A posterior interosseous artery flap may be possible with smaller wounds. A groin flap is always a good lifeboat option. Some surgeons advocate proceeding directly to a free microvascular transfer of tissue to prevent the hand from being connected to the groin.

Principles and Clinical Pearls

- The dorsal skin is thin, and any flap used should optimally match this quality as closely as possible.
- The need for further treatment, including extensor tenolysis and extensor tendon grafting, must be anticipated at the time of flap transfer.
- The radial forearm fascia flap provides optimal re-creation of the thin skin; however, more durable flaps may be necessary.

Pitfalls

Flap loss can occur if the radial artery flow is inadequate. Thicker flaps may create a biscuit phenomenon, in which the thick dorsal skin requires multiple defatting procedures. Extensor tendon scarring and metacarpophalangeal joint scarring will lead to significant hand dysfunction. These joints and tendons need to be addressed.

Classic References

Ho AM, Chang J. Radial artery perforator flap. J Hand Surg Am 35:308, 2010.
The radial artery perforator flap was discussed. In this flap, the radial artery does not need to be sacrificed.

Page R, Chang J. Reconstruction of hand soft-tissue defects: alternatives to the radial forearm fasciocutaneous flap. J Hand Surg Am 31:847, 2006.
Several alternatives to the radial forearm fasciocutaneous flap were proposed that will lead to better tailoring of the reconstruction.

Rehim SA, Singhal M, Chung KC. Dermal skin substitutes for upper limb reconstruction: current status, indications, and contraindications. Hand Clin 30:239, 2014.
Dermal skin substitutes were discussed as alternatives for coverage of exposed tendons.

63 Paint-Gun Injection Injury

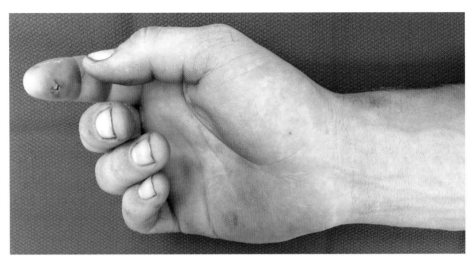

This 32-year-old construction worker had a paint-injection injury while cleaning the nozzle of his injector. He is seen in the emergency department 2 hours after the injury, with a pinpoint wound on his right index fingertip and swelling of his entire finger.

Description of the Problem

Paint-gun injuries typically occur while the operator is trying to clear a blocked nozzle or steady the gun with the free hand. High-pressure grease and paint guns can generate pressures of up to 12,000 psi. Significant tissue necrosis can occur, depending on the type of paint. Oil-based paint is worse than grease, which in turn is worse than latex and water-based paint. The potential severity of high-pressure injection injuries is underappreciated; as a result, they are often misdiagnosed. Although frequently only a small pinpoint wound occurs on the fingertip, the high-pressure injection can spread paint proximally along soft tissue planes. The injected materials dissect proximally along the neurovascular bundles and the flexor tendon sheath into the hand.

Key Anatomy

The neurovascular bundles and flexor tendon tunnels are "highways" that allow spread of the paint, grease, or other high-pressure-injected material into the hand. The resulting inflammation within the tight confines of the finger may cause digital ischemia. The injected material is trapped within the soft tissues and can impregnate the digital nerves, arteries, and tendons.

Workup

Patients should be prepared urgently for debridement in the operating room. Plain radiographs may show the extent of the paint spread if the paint has a lead content. The only reliable way to appreciate the extent of spread within the tissues is by direct surgical exploration.

Treatment

The finger and palm are opened widely using either Bruner zigzag incisions or an extensile midaxial incision carried into the palm by zigzag extensions. Meticulous debridement and copious irrigation are carried out to remove as much injected material as possible. Pulse lavage irrigation is contraindicated. The flexor tendon sheath is opened, and the A2 and A4 pulleys are preserved. Necrotic skin at the site of injection is debrided. The digital neurovascular bundles should be isolated, cleaned, and preserved. The hand is explored in a distal to proximal direction until normal tissue planes are found. Intravenous antibiotics and tetanus prophylaxis are given. The benefits of intravenous corticosteroids are unproven. A second-look operation may be required. Soft tissue coverage procedures in the form of cross-finger flaps, heterodigital island flaps, distant fasciocutaneous flaps, and skin grafts may be required. Even with appropriate treatment, the finger may eventually need amputation.

Alternatives

There are no treatment alternatives. This is an operative case that should be taken to surgery as soon as possible.

Principles and Clinical Pearls

- Paint-gun injection injuries are underappreciated.
- Urgent exploration, irrigation, and debridement are warranted, however small the wound. Operative exploration proceeds until normal tissue is found.
- The extent of tissue injury is dependent on the pressure of injection, the type and amount of paint, and the time from injection to debridement.

Pitfalls

Failure to recognize this injury will lead to extensive tissue necrosis in the finger and possibly the hand. Amputation of the finger or the ray may be required. Patients should not be discharged from the hospital without undergoing a formal exploration in the operating room.

Classic References

Amsdell SL, Hammert WC. High-pressure injection injuries in the hand: current treatment concepts. Plast Reconstr Surg 132:586e, 2013.
This most-recent review acknowledges that the literature is filled only with case reports and small series of cases because of the relative rarity of the injury. No randomized trials are published. However, interesting combined data are available on the relative risks of amputation, depending on the material injected and the time to treatment.

Gelberman RH, Posch JL, Jurist JM. High-pressure injection injuries of the hand. J Bone Joint Surg Am 57:935, 1975.
In this series of 26 patients, the authors found that the most commonly injected materials were automotive grease, diesel oil, and paint. Paint injections, especially into the digits, did poorly and often resulted in digital amputation. The total disability after amputation was related directly to the time elapsed between the initial injury and the amputation. The authors concluded: "Although we were unable to specifically relate the ultimate result to the time elapsed between injury and proper treatment, we continue to recommend early, aggressive, wide debridement of these injuries."

Lozano-Calderón SA, Mudgal CS, Mudgal S, Ring D. Latex paint-gun injuries of the hand: are the outcomes better? Hand (N Y) 3:340, 2008.
In this series of five patients, the authors attributed the excellent outcomes to the type of paint—latex-based rather than oil-based—that was injected. They also highlighted the importance of prompt management for this seemingly innocuous injury.

Instability

64 Ulnar Collateral Ligament Tear of the Thumb Metacarpophalangeal Joint

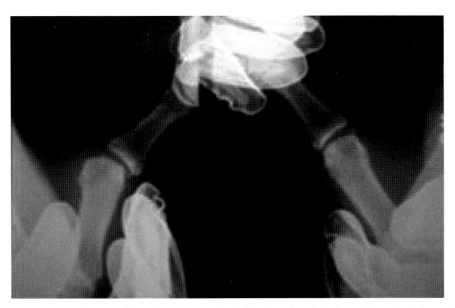

This 22-year-old skier fell on her outstretched right hand and abducted thumb during a downhill ski run. She had immediate pain along the ulnar aspect of her thumb metacarpophalangeal (MCP) joint and was unable to hold a key or zip her ski jacket afterward. On a physical examination the next day, she had substantial bruising at the ulnar aspect of the MCP joint. A palpable mass was present ulnar to the neck of her thumb metacarpal. She was tender to palpation of the ulnar aspect of the base of her proximal phalanx. Gentle radial stress of the thumb using the MCP joint as a fulcrum provoked pain and instability. A stress radiograph of the MCP joints is shown.

Description of the Problem

Avulsion of the thumb MCP ulnar collateral ligament (UCL) is a common injury in younger patients. With forcible hyperabduction of the thumb at the MCP joint, the ligament avulses from the base of the proximal phalanx and remains attached to the head of the metacarpal. The ligament ruptures in its midportion infrequently. Occasionally, an avulsion fracture of the base of the proximal phalanx is present. The proximal, leading edge of the adductor pollicis aponeurosis can trap the avulsed ligament proximally (and superficially). Ligament-to-bone healing is impossible in the absence of surgical treatment to restore the ligament deep to the adductor aponeurosis, adjacent to its insertion on the base of the proximal phalanx. Differential diagnosis includes fracture of the metacarpal or the proximal phalanx, a radial collateral ligament tear, and a dorsoradial capsular avulsion.

Key Anatomy

A direct dorsoulnar surgical approach is used to repair the UCL avulsion. A dorsal cutaneous branch of the radial sensory nerve is present directly on the extensor tendons and retinacular attachments. This should be sought specifically and protected. The adductor aponeurosis is identified, and a soft tissue mass projecting superficially proximal to the aponeurosis is a so-called Stener lesion of the UCL. This is frequently slightly hemorrhagic and represents the distal end of the avulsed UCL. Retraction or transection (followed by repair) of the adductor aponeurosis is needed for exposure of the ulnar aspect of the base of the proximal phalanx for direct ligament repair.

Workup

PA and lateral plain radiographs of the thumb base are needed for an initial diagnosis of a fracture. Stress radiographs (see the figure) are used to demonstrate proximal phalangeal translation on the head of the metacarpal. This finding indicates MCP instability. The thumb is evaluated in full extension and in 30 degrees of flexion to assess the proper UCL and the accessory UCL separately. An MRI can be obtained to assess for ligament tear or displacement.

Treatment

Surgical repair of the thumb UCL is critical. The presence of an avulsion-type fracture of the thumb proximal phalanx is not, in itself, an indication for surgery, because the thumb MCP joint can be stable to radial stress even in the presence of this type of fracture. If the thumb is stable to radial stress, then casting for 4 to 6 weeks should be sufficient. After surgical reattachment of the UCL to the base of the proximal phalanx (with an intraosseous suture anchor), the joint can be pinned for 4 to 6 weeks to allow initial healing. This is done at the surgeon's discretion. The thumb is immobilized in a cast after the surgical repair.

Alternatives

Acute injuries with Stener lesions are treated by operative repair, whereas acute injuries without Stener lesions can be immobilized until they heal (as long as they do not exhibit valgus stress of greater than 35 degrees while the MCP is held in full extension). Proximal phalanx base fractures with associated instability are treated operatively, whereas fractures without instability can be treated operatively if joint incongruity is substantial. Chronic injuries without arthritis can be treated nonoperatively; however, the UCL can be surgically reconstructed or the MCP joint can be arthrodesed. Chronic injuries with arthritis are treated by MCP joint arthrodesis.

Principles and Clinical Pearls

- The radial sensory nerve should always be identified during the initial surgical approach.
- Pinning of the MCP joint is not required but is preferred by many surgeons to allow ligament healing to bone.
- Either valgus stress opening to more than 35 degrees (at full MCP extension) or proximal phalangeal translation radially over the metacarpal head can be used to radiographically diagnose an operative tear.

Pitfalls

Complications of surgical treatment include persistent instability as a result of impaired ligament-bone healing. Other complications include radial sensory nerve injury and pin tract infection (and possible septic arthritis).

Classic Reference

Heyman P, Gelberman RH, Duncan K, Hipp JA. Injuries of the ulnar collateral ligament of the thumb metacarpophalangeal joint. Biomechanical and prospective clinical studies on the usefulness of valgus stress testing. Clin Orthop Relat Res 292:165, 1993.

Proper collateral ligament transection alone resulted in MCP joint laxity at 30 degrees of flexion. When the accessory collateral ligament was also transected, laxity was demonstrated in full MCP extension. Clinically, greater than 35 degrees of valgus angulation during stress testing indicated the presence of both proper collateral and accessory collateral tears. Stener lesions were present in 87% of these cases.

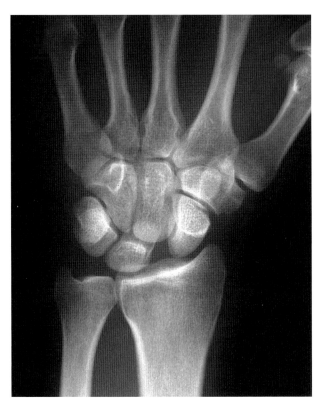

This 23-year-old woman presents to her primary care doctor 2 weeks after a fall onto her outstretched wrist while playing soccer. She had immediate pain over the dorsoradial aspect of her wrist; however, she thought it was just a sprain and continued to play. After 2 weeks, the pain and swelling have not resolved. She has weakness, pain, and swelling over the radial aspect of the dorsal wrist. She has limited range of passive and active flexion of the wrist and point tenderness 1 cm distal to the Lister tubercle. No other sites of point tenderness are noted on examination. A Watson test (dorsal-directed pressure on the volar scaphoid tubercle while moving the hand and wrist from a position of radial deviation to ulnar deviation and assessing for pain and a palpable "clunk") is positive. A PA radiograph of the wrist is shown. (Photo courtesy of Richard Gelberman, MD.)

Description of the Problem

Complete tears of the scapholunate ligament can present acutely; however, they are infrequently appreciated after they occur initially, and presentation is often delayed, sometimes for weeks or months. The scaphoid assumes an obligate position of flexion, and the lunate, no longer tethered to the scaphoid through the scapholunate ligament, assumes a position of obligate extension. This static carpal instability pattern leads to a recognizable pattern of radiocarpal and intercarpal arthritis and will cause pain, motion loss, and decreased strength.

Key Anatomy

The scapholunate interosseous ligament is strongest dorsally, whereas the lunotriquetral ligament is strongest volarly. Along with the scaphotrapeziotrapezoid capsule and ligaments and the extrinsic volar radioscaphocapitate ligament, these capsuloligamentous restraints maintain the scaphoid in relative extension and allow composite wrist motion along the extension–radial deviation and the flexion–ulnar deviation arc.

Workup

PA, lateral, PA ulnar deviation, and supinated clench fist (neutral flexion-extension) radiographs are obtained. If necessary, comparison views of the contralateral, normal side are obtained. MRI arthrography can help to confirm the diagnosis if the extent of the tear or the presence of a concomitant lunotriquetral ligament tear is questionable.

Treatment

Open reduction, ligament repair, and scapholunate pinning (with or without scaphocapitate pinning) are recommended if treatment is possible within 3 weeks of the injury. After this time, the results of this approach can be less reliable in restoring the normal position of scaphoid extension and scapholunate congruity. A dorsal surgical approach through the third dorsal extensor compartment can allow access to the ligament and facilitate direct anatomic reduction using joysticks and a ligament repair using suture anchors. For a delayed repair, some authors advocate a capsulodesis, combined with a ligament repair, to provide a static restraint to scaphoid flexion. This treatment will limit active and passive wrist flexion, but can prevent arthritic degeneration of the radiocarpal joint.

Alternatives

Patients with a delayed presentation can undergo tendoligamentous reconstruction using the flexor carpi radialis tendon or static capsulodesis procedures with or without a radial styloidectomy. Nonoperative treatment is an option in these patients, because there is no universal consensus that arthritis, pain, and limitation of motion are inevitable after such treatment. For treatment of a chronic scapholunate ligament tear, salvage options include a four-corner arthrodesis with a scaphoid excision, a proximal-row carpectomy, a wrist arthrodesis, and a total wrist arthroplasty.

Principles and Clinical Pearls

- For injuries less than 3 weeks old, empiric data and observation suggest that open reduction and pinning of the scapholunate and the scaphocapitate joints are of benefit in an attempt to influence ligament healing.
- Early radiography and MRI should be performed if a scapholunate ligament tear is suspected, and surgical treatment should not be delayed if the diagnosis is confirmed.
- A dorsal surgical approach through the third dorsal compartment allows access to the scaphoid, the lunate, and the scapholunate ligament.
- Some surgeons advocate temporary intra-operative pinning of the lunate to the radius to decrease the difficulty in achieving an anatomic reduction of the scapholunate articulation.

Pitfalls

Removal of the pin too early (before 8 weeks) does not allow sufficient time for ligament healing and can result in failure of surgical treatment. As with scaphoid fractures, the missed diagnosis continues to be a problem and will bedevil future surgeons unless the diagnosis is made with alacrity and surgical treatment initiated before it is too late.

Classic Reference

Watson HK, Ballet FL. The SLAC wrist: scapholunate advanced collapse pattern of degenerative arthritis. J Hand Surg Am 9:358, 1984.
This article was the first to describe the reproducible and recognizable pattern of posttraumatic radiocarpal and intercarpal arthritis that develops after a scapholunate ligament tear.

66 Sagittal Band Rupture

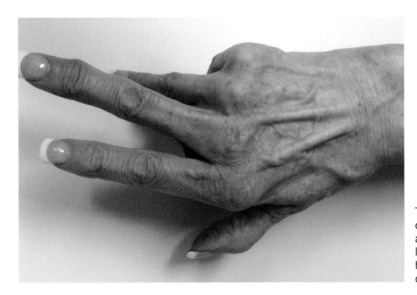

This 60-year-old woman has developed locking of her right index and middle finger metacarpophalangeal (MCP) joints with flexion of her fingers while making a fist. This causes discomfort.

Description of the Problem

On examination, the patient has subluxation of the index and middle finger extensor tendons ulnarly while making a fist. She has disruption of the radial sagittal bands to these fingers over the dorsum of the MCP joints.

Key Anatomy

As the extrinsic extensor tendon passes over the metacarpal head, it is stabilized in a central position by the sagittal band on either side. The fibers of the sagittal bands come from the extensor tendons and pass around the metacarpal head on the radial and ulnar sides to insert onto the volar plate. These bands ensure centralization of the extensor tendon over the apex of the metacarpal head as the tendon glides over the joint. Because the radial sagittal bands have ruptured in this patient, the extensor tendons have slipped off the apex ulnarly and lost their central position and mechanical advantage.

Workup

A history of possible trauma should be reviewed. In patients with multiple sagittal band ruptures, a rheumatologic evaluation should be undertaken. Closed sagittal band injuries are often seen in patients with rheumatoid arthritis. A radiograph is obtained to rule out MCP joint arthritis and subluxation. The volar side is evaluated for evidence of a trigger finger, which would cause a popping with flexion.

Treatment

When diagnosed within the first 2 to 3 weeks after an injury, sagittal band ruptures may possibly be treated conservatively with a splinting of the MCP joint in full extension. The PIP joint should remain free to allow active motion. However, direct repair of a late sagittal band rupture is usually not possible, because the sagittal band has contracted. Late reconstruction requires some additional tendon repair around the region. For this purpose, juncturae tendinum or a proximally or distally based portion of the extensor tendon itself may be dissected and used to suture from the remaining extensor hood to around the lumbrical tendon. This tendon graft reconstruction needs to be carefully protected for several weeks before active flexion exercises are initiated.

Alternatives

Alternatives for tendon reconstruction of the sagittal band include the use of a free tendon graft from the palmaris longus tendon or another tendon donor. Patients may choose to not have a procedure once they are counseled on the imperfections.

Principles and Clinical Pearls

- The differential diagnosis for an inability to extend the MCP joint includes radial nerve palsy, sagittal band rupture, MCP joint subluxation, and trigger finger. These can be differentiated based on the history and physical examination.
- A rheumatologic workup is critical in patients with multiple sagittal band ruptures.
- In cases of chronic sagittal band rupture, the use of juncturae tendinum or a portion of the extensor tendon itself is useful to re-create a sagittal band.

Pitfalls

The main pitfall of any late reconstruction is recurrence of the sagittal band rupture and dislocation of the extensor tendon. Patients can have difficulty with full flexion at the MCP joint if the tension is too tight. Last, over time, a sagittal band rupture may recur with activity.

Classic References

Peelman J, Markiewitz A, Kiefhaber T, Stern P. Splintage in the treatment of sagittal band incompetence and extensor tendon subluxation. J Hand Surg Eur Vol 40:287, 2015.
This article presented a retrospective review of patients treated with splinting for sagittal band rupture. Acute and sub-acute injuries were amenable to splinting. Splinting proved very effective for these early injuries. This highlighted the need for early recognition.

Watson H, Weinzweig J, Guidera PM. Sagittal band reconstruction. J Hand Surg Am 22:452, 1997.
This paper was written in 1997 and continues to be an excellent article, describing the technique of weaving a retrograde segment of extensor tendon for reconstruction of a sagittal band.

Osteonecrosis

67 Kienböck Disease

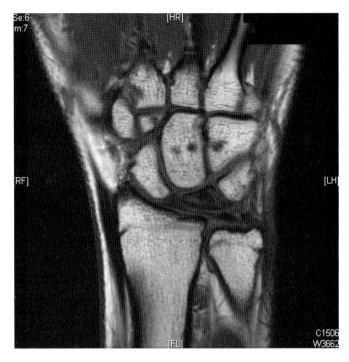

This is an MRI scan of a 16-year-old girl with pain in her right wrist. She presents for an evaluation.

Description of the Problem

The MRI shows decreased flow to the lunate, which seems to be collapsed. The patient may have Kienböck disease. Although the classification of this disease is based on radiographic findings, the patient probably has stage 3A disease.

Key Anatomy

Kienböck disease is an idiopathic avascular necrosis of the lunate bone. This bone occupies an important place in the proximal row, because it prevents proximal migration of the capitate. The cause of Kienböck disease is unknown; over time, decreased blood flow to the lunate leads to progressive collapse. The architecture of the remaining carpal bones is disturbed, and progressive arthritis develops. The length of the radius, compared with that of the ulna, is critical. Ulnar negative variance is implicated in the cause of the disease, because the radius places undue pressure on the lunate.

Workup

Chronic wrist pain of any cause warrants a careful examination for masses or instability in the wrist. Radiographs are obtained first. In this case, the radiograph shows sclerosis of the lunate (with a more whitened lunate) and/or collapse of the lunate's height. The radiograph should be carefully assessed for ulnar negative variance as a predisposing factor to Kienböck disease. Usually, an MRI is obtained to assess blood flow to the lunate. Decreased flow to the lunate is diagnostic for Kienböck disease.

Treatment

The treatment for Kienböck disease is based on the Lichtman classification scheme, which is determined with radiographs. In stage 1, radiographs are normal, and revascularization can be performed with a vascularized bone graft, typically from the 3, 4 extracompartmental artery. This is also true for stage II disease, in which sclerosis of the lunate is present without the collapse. For stage 1 and 2, if ulnar negative variance is evident, the radius can be shortened with a radial osteotomy. In stage 3A, the lunate has avascular necrosis, collapse, and fragmentation, and the capitate has migrated proximally. Stage 3B has the same findings as those of stage 3A, with a flexion deformity of the scaphoid. The optimal treatment for this stage is a topic of debate—some surgeons prefer a radial shortening with or without vascularized bone graft, whereas others proceed directly to a proximal-row carpectomy or scaphotrapeziotrapezoidal fusion. In stage 4, collapse of the lunate is accompanied by radiocarpal and midcarpal arthrosis on radiographs. In this case, the lunate cannot be salvaged, and if pain is worsening, the best treatment is wrist fusion.

This patient probably has stage 3A Kienböck disease. Even though the lunate is a bit collapsed, we would advocate performing a radial shortening osteotomy and then attempting a vascularized bone graft from the 3, 4 extracompartmental artery. The lunate may be opened and expanded to receive the bone graft. At the same time, the posterior interosseous nerve is transected to decrease pain to the wrist.

Alternatives

In this case of stage 3A Kienböck disease, the debate is whether to perform a reconstructive procedure consisting of a radial osteotomy and vascularized bone graft or whether to proceed directly to a proximal-row carpectomy. Another option that has been advocated to unload the lunate is a capitate shortening.

Principles and Clinical Pearls

- In cases of chronic wrist pain centered over the lunate, a radiograph and MRI are critical to evaluate for avascular necrosis of the lunate.
- The Lichtman classification scheme is excellent, because it is useful for determining treatment based on the radiographic findings.
- The treatment of Kienböck disease is based on two concepts. The first is to unload the proximal row by either capitate shortening or radial shortening, and the second is to revascularize the lunate.

Pitfalls

The treatment of Kienböck disease is unlikely to restore full range of painless motion. All the procedures described are performed in an attempt to salvage an essentially dead bone; therefore they may not be successful, and salvage operations may be necessary in the future. Furthermore, all of these surgeries will decrease the range of motion of the wrist.

Classic Reference

Matsui Y, Funakoshi T, Motomiya M, Urita A, Minami M, Iwasaki N. Radial shortening osteotomy for Kienböck disease: minimum 10-year follow-up. J Hand Surg Am 39:679, 2014.
A radial shortening osteotomy is a common procedure for treating Kienböck disease. This was a review of one center's experience with radial shortening.

Peripheral Nerve

68 Carpal Tunnel Syndrome

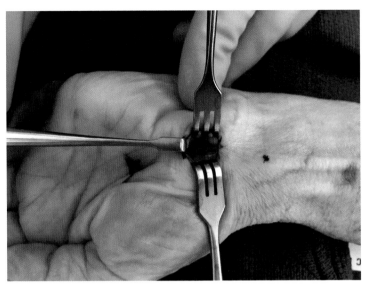

This 48-year-old surgeon presented to his primary care doctor's office with numbness and tingling over the volar aspect of his thumb, index, and middle fingers and the radial aspect of his ring finger. The tingling woke him up twice every night and was made worse by driving, typing on his portable computer, and donning gloves for surgery. He had tried wearing resting wrist splints, but they did not help. He was otherwise healthy except for gastroesophageal reflux. On an examination, he had a positive Tinel sign bilaterally, a positive Durkan sign, and a positive Phalen test. His two-point discrimination was 5 mm in the middle finger and 2 to 3 mm in all other fingers. He had no thenar atrophy, but mild weakness on strength testing was noted. He had no proximal Tinel sign over the pronator teres muscle and no Tinel sign over the ulnar nerve in the cubital tunnel. A Spurling test was negative.

Description of the Problem

Carpal tunnel syndrome is caused by median nerve compression as it passes deep to the transverse carpal ligament in the carpal tunnel. Although it can be caused by masses within the carpal tunnel (such as a tumor or hematoma), infection, synovitis, or trauma, it is most frequently idiopathic. A differential diagnosis includes C6 radiculopathy, proximal compression of the median nerve beneath the leading edge of the pronator teres muscle, and other causes of mononeuritides.

Key Anatomy

The carpal tunnel is bounded superiorly by the undersurface of the transverse carpal ligament, on the deep aspect by the anterior aspect of the capitate and the lunate, radially by the trapezium and the scaphoid, and ulnarly by the triquetrum, the hamate, and the pisiform. It contains the nine digital flexor tendons (four flexor digitorum superficialis tendons, four flexor digitorum profundus tendons, and one flexor pollicis longus tendon) and the median nerve. The median nerve is typically located just deep to the transverse carpal ligament on the radial aspect of the carpal tunnel. The palmar cutaneous branch of the median nerve is located superficial to the transverse carpal ligament immediately ulnar to the flexor carpi radialis tendon, and the recurrent motor branch of the median nerve emanates most often from the radial, volar-radial, or the volar aspect of the median nerve distally in the carpal tunnel. Cutaneous landmarks that aid in the planning of incisions include the hook of the hamate (denoting the radialmost aspect of Guyon canal and the ulnar neurovascular bundle) and the flexor carpi radialis tendon (whose ulnar aspect marks the location of the palmar cutaneous branch of the median nerve as it crosses the wrist crease).

Workup

Electrophysiologic assessment in the form of nerve conduction velocity testing (to assess for increased motor latency) or electromyography (to assess for signs of thenar muscle denervation) can be used to good effect, although not all surgeons think that it is required before surgical treatment.

Treatment

Nonoperative treatments that have been advocated include oral antiinflammatory drugs, splinting of the wrist in neutral position (sometimes for 24 hours/day), and a direct intracarpal canal injection of corticosteroid formulations. Although splinting has been shown to be useful in mild cases in which no objective sensory or motor loss is detected, and steroid injection has been shown to have positive short-term effects for a month to a year, the benchmark treatment of this condition is decompression of the carpal tunnel by dividing the transverse carpal ligament. In a typical open carpal tunnel release, the transverse carpal ligament is divided on its ulnar aspect, and release is carried distally (until yellow fat that surrounds the superficial palmar arterial arch is visible) and proximally (until complete release of the proximal aspect of the transverse carpal ligament and the distal aspect of the volar antebrachial fascia is seen).

Alternatives

Open, limited open, and endoscopic techniques have been advocated. Although some studies have intimated that endoscopic release can lead to a shortened recovery time and better patient tolerance of the procedure and its recovery, most surgeons favor open release for its reliability, low complication rate, and reproducibility of results. Corticosteroid injections can be used to temporize until the patient is able to undergo a surgical procedure. It can also be used in patients with a primary inflammatory process of the carpal tunnel and in pregnant or postpartum women who wish to postpone or decline surgical treatment.

Principles and Clinical Pearls

- Concurrent C6 radiculopathy is common, and this "double-crush" phenomenon can lead to incomplete relief after a successful release of the transverse carpal ligament.
- An ulnar approach to the transverse carpal ligament can minimize the risk of damage to the palmar cutaneous branch of the median nerve and to the recurrent motor branch of the median nerve. Too-vigorous retraction of the ulnar soft tissues superficial to the transverse carpal ligament can result in ulnar nerve irritation.
- Additional surgical treatment of carpal tunnel syndrome in the form of external or internal neurolysis has not been shown to be of value, even in cases with demonstrable electrophysiologic or physical evidence of axonal loss.

Pitfalls

Patient dissatisfaction after carpal tunnel release can be attributed to a failure of diagnosis (an incorrect preoperative diagnosis), a failure of surgical treatment (an incomplete release of the ligament, the median nerve injury, or a laceration), or postoperative complications or difficulty (a painful scar, pillar pain, an infection, or wound dehiscence). A careful history of preoperative signs and symptoms and the timing of postoperative signs and symptoms can help in differentiating these conditions.

Classic Reference

Gelberman RH, Pfeffer GB, Galbraith RT, Szabo RM, Rydevik B, Dimick M. Results of treatment of severe carpal-tunnel syndrome without internal neurolysis of the median nerve. J Bone Joint Surg Am 69:896, 1987.

This was one of many papers from this author and his colleagues that demonstrated the futility of additional surgical machinations in the treatment of this common condition. Simply stated, release of the transverse carpal ligament is all that is ever required for the surgical treatment of this condition.

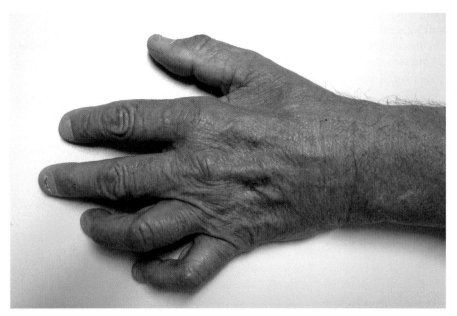

This 55-year-old man presents with a 6-month history of left hand weakness and numbness. He is unable to hold a pen or a key normally and notices that his hand feels clumsy, especially during fine motor activity. He is unable to button his shirt or pants and has noted an inability to cross and uncross his fingers. His physical examination reveals wasting of the first dorsal interosseous muscle, an inability to execute key pinch without keeping his thumb interphalangeal joint flexed (a positive Froment sign), an inability to adduct his small finger when the metacarpophalangeal joint is held in full extension (a Wartenburg sign), an inability to extend the proximal interphalangeal and distal interphalangeal joints of his small and ring fingers while the metacarpophalangeal joints are in full extension (clawing), weak flexion of the distal interphalangeal joints of the small and ring fingers, and lancinating pain and tingling when the ulnar nerve is percussed behind the medial epicondyle (a Tinel sign). A sensory examination demonstrates decreased sensation over the dorsovolar aspects of the ulnar metacarpus and increased static two-point discrimination over the ulnar aspect of the ring finger pulp and the radial and ulnar aspects of the small finger pulp.

Description of the Problem

Cubital tunnel syndrome is a descriptive term for ulnar nerve entrapment about the elbow. Nerve compression can occur proximally at the arcade of Struthers, deep to Osborne's fascia posterior to the medial epicondyle, between the two heads of the flexor carpi ulnaris muscle, and deep to the fascia overlying the flexor digitorum profundus muscle. A differential diagnosis includes C7, C8, or T1 radiculopathy; amyotrophic lateral sclerosis; a Pancoast tumor; shingles; a brachial plexus lesion (the lower trunk or medial cord); a Guyon canal compression; and an ulnar artery aneurysm or thrombosis.

Key Anatomy

The course of the ulnar nerve in the distal arm and the proximal forearm determines the sites of compression of the nerve mentioned previously. After transposition of the ulnar nerve anteriorly, the medial intermuscular septum can be a site of compression if it is not resected at surgery.

Workup

A workup includes electrophysiologic assessment to measure ulnar nerve conduction velocity across the elbow (a drop in velocity of 20% or a difference from the contralateral side of 15 meters/sec, although these values are not accepted universally) and electromyography of ulnar nerve–innervated muscles to evaluate for denervation. In patients with a history of elbow trauma or elbow deformity, PA and lateral plain radiographs of the elbow should be obtained.

Treatment

Splinting the elbow in 50 degrees of flexion minimizes intrinsic ulnar nerve pressure and might increase intraneural blood flow. Operative treatment involves decompression of the ulnar nerve at the cubital tunnel either with or without anterior transposition (subcutaneous, intramuscular, or submuscular) and with or without a medial epicondylectomy. The medial intermuscular septum should be resected if the nerve is transposed.

Alternatives

There are no treatment alternatives.

Principles and Clinical Pearls

- Rule out all other potential sites of cervical nerve root, lower trunk, medial cord, and ulnar nerve compression, including distal compression in the Guyon canal.
- Motor weakness with a normal sensory examination should prompt investigation for motor neuron disease.
- The medial antebrachial cutaneous nerve lies on the enveloping fascia of the forearm and should be sought and protected during exposure of the medial elbow. Injury to this nerve causes paresthesias posterior to the incision and a type 2 complex regional pain syndrome from neuroma development.

Pitfalls

Pitfalls include an ulnar nerve injury (neurapraxia, axonotmesis, or neurotmesis), recurrence or persistence of symptoms, a medial antebrachial nerve injury (neurapraxia, axonotmesis, or neurotmesis), an incorrect or incomplete diagnosis, wound dehiscence, a hematoma, and a fixed flexion deformity of the elbow.

Classic Reference

Gelberman RH, Eaton RG, Urbaniak JR. Peripheral nerve compression. Instr Course Lect 43:31, 1994.
This useful review article covered the anatomy, pathophysiology, and surgical treatment of three common nerve compression syndromes: carpal tunnel syndrome, cubital tunnel syndrome, and radial tunnel syndrome.

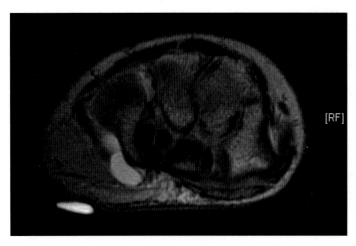

This 42-year-old patient presents with ulnar nerve intrinsic muscle paralysis and a palpable mass at the base of the wrist in the region of the Guyon canal. In this axial MRI scan at the level of the wrist, the marker outside the skin designates the area of the mass. Adjacent to the hook of the hamate, a fluid structure is compressing the ulnar nerve and artery.

Description of the Problem

A fluid-filled structure in the Guyon canal is most likely a ganglion that is compressing the motor branch of the ulnar nerve.

Key Anatomy

The ulnar nerve proceeds distally in the distal forearm into the Guyon canal. This canal is a tight space between the pisiform ulnarly and the hook of the hamate radially. The ulnar nerve branches into the deep motor branch and the superficial sensory branches. The ulnar artery courses through this area and then forms the superficial arch.

Workup

A patient with a Guyon tunnel mass is likely to present with isolated ulnar nerve intrinsic weakness or atrophy of the ulnar innervated muscles. These muscles include the first dorsal interosseous muscle and the hypothenar muscles, which are easily palpated. The patient will have difficulty abducting and adducting his fingers and weakness of pinch. In a patient with isolated ulnar intrinsic weakness or paralysis, causes of compression or injury to the motor branch of the ulnar nerve should be suspected. The Guyon canal is a very tight space; therefore any space-occupying lesion may compress the ulnar motor branch.

The classic diagnosis is a ganglion that emanates from the pisotriquetral joint. Radiographs should be obtained to rule out a hook of hamate fracture (see Chapter 53). Special carpal tunnel views may be necessary to find the hook of hamate fracture. Most important, an MRI scan should be performed to both rule out the hook of hamate fracture and to assess for a space-occupying lesion such as a ganglion.

Treatment

In patients with a ganglion in the Guyon canal, a Guyon tunnel release and excision of the ganglion are critical. Dissection in this region must be performed very carefully. The ulnar nerve should be first identified proximally in the distal wrist and then followed as the Guyon canal is opened. The ulnar artery is protected, and the ulnar nerve is carefully dissected to identify the motor branch of the ulnar nerve. The mass is excised, and all branches of the ulnar nerve are preserved.

Alternatives

The best treatment is surgical excision of the mass. The ganglion should not be aspirated, because the ulnar artery or ulnar nerve could be directly injured in this tight space. Surgery should not be delayed in patients with ulnar nerve paralysis or weakness.

Principles and Clinical Pearls

- The Guyon canal contains the ulnar artery and ulnar nerve, both of which are essential for hand function.
- The deep branch of the ulnar nerve is a critical nerve because of the extensive number of ulnar-innervated intrinsic muscles.
- A ganglion in the Guyon canal should be suspected in any case of ulnar nerve paralysis distally.

Pitfalls

Pitfalls are related to injury to the motor branch of the ulnar nerve. This nerve is at risk in any procedure in the Guyon canal, including a ganglion excision, a hook of hamate excision, and an ulnar artery surgery. Low ulnar nerve palsy is very difficult to correct with tendon transfers and other salvage procedures.

Classic References

Maroukis BL, Ogawa T, Rehim SA, Chung KC. Guyon canal: the evolution of clinical anatomy. J Hand Surg Am 40:560, 2015.
This article was very interesting, because it discussed the history of Dr. Guyon and the original anatomic descriptions and controversies regarding clinical associations of the Guyon canal.

Wang B, Zhao Y, Lu A, Chen C. Ulnar nerve deep branch compression by a ganglion: a review of nine cases. Injury 45:1126, 2014.
Even though a ganglion in the Guyon canal is a well-known clinical entity, case series are rare. This was a fairly large series of nine cases of compression of the deep motor branch of the ulnar nerve by a ganglion.

Xing SG, Tang JB. Entrapment neuropathy of the wrist, forearm, and elbow. Clin Plast Surg 41:561, 2014.
This was an excellent overview of all entrapment neuropathies in the wrist, forearm, and elbow, including ulnar nerve compression at the wrist, otherwise known as ulnar tunnel syndrome.

71 Radial Tunnel Syndrome

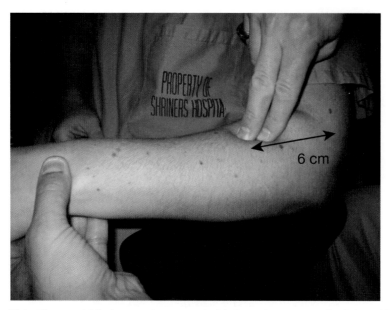

6 cm

This 40-year-old factory worker presented to her primary care physician with a 2-month history of pain in her left, nondominant elbow and proximal forearm. The patient described daily repetitive work. She localized the pain to the proximal radial forearm. She has had difficulty removing a gallon of milk from the refrigerator and lifting objects weighing more than 3 pounds. Antiinflammatory medications have provided little relief. On a physical examination, the patient has point tenderness over the proximal radius just ulnar to the mobile wad musculature and point tenderness on the radial side (posterior aspect) of the mobile wad just over the radial shaft approximately 10 cm distal to the elbow. She has no tenderness over the lateral epicondyle and no tenderness contralaterally. A counterforce brace has provided no relief.

Description of the Problem

Radial tunnel syndrome is a compression of the radial nerve in the proximal forearm. It can occur simultaneously with lateral tennis elbow syndrome.

Key Anatomy

The radial nerve passes into the proximal forearm between the brachialis and the brachioradialis. As it enters the proximodorsal forearm, it passes deep to fibrous bands proximal to the extensor muscle origin, then passes deep to, in order: the recurrent leash of Henry, the extensor carpi radialis origin, the aponeurosis at the leading edge of the supinator muscle, and the supinator muscle. It exits the supinator muscle as the posterior interosseous nerve. It is generally accepted that the radial wrist extensor muscles are supplied by the radial nerve, and the digital and thumb extensors and abductor pollicis longus are supplied by the posterior interosseous nerve. The supinator is supplied either by the radial nerve or by early branches of the posterior interosseous nerve. The most commonly described site of compression of the radial nerve in radial tunnel syndrome is at the leading edge of the supinator (the arcade of Frohse).

Workup

No workup is needed. Electrophysiologic testing is usually not helpful in diagnosing radial tunnel syndrome.

176

Treatment

Antiinflammatory medications, wrist splints, and activity modification have been advocated; however, none has been shown to reliably treat this condition. Surgical treatment is by decompression of the radial tunnel either from an anterior or a posterior approach to the radial nerve and the posterior interosseous nerve in the proximal forearm. The compression points noted previously are addressed. Accessing the proximal aspect of the radial tunnel from a posterior approach is difficult, as is accessing the distal aspect of the radial tunnel from the anterior approach.

Alternatives

Some question the validity of this condition as a diagnosis separate from lateral tennis elbow syndrome. Plain radiographs or an MRI can help to differentiate idiopathic radial tunnel syndrome from a mass lesion in the proximal forearm causing either motor loss or sensory symptoms of the posterior interosseous nerve and the radial nerve.

Principles and Clinical Pearls

- Radial tunnel syndrome is a clinical diagnosis.
- Modifying a patient's specific work activity is always easier than surgical treatment.
- Accessing the entire radial tunnel through a single incision, either anterior or posterior, is difficult.

Pitfalls

Radial tunnel syndrome is a pain syndrome. Conversely, posterior interosseous nerve compression is a motor neuropathy that can be evaluated by electromyography. Radial nerve injury in the arm leads to both motor and sensory symptoms in the radial nerve distribution. Whether compression of the radial nerve or of the posterior interosseous nerve in the proximal forearm (as in radial tunnel syndrome) leads to a pain syndrome rather than definable motor or sensory findings is a part of the debate regarding the authenticity of this as a definable condition.

Classic Reference

Urch EY, Model Z, Wolfe SW, Lee SK. Anatomical study of the surgical approaches to the radial tunnel. J Hand Surg Am 40:1416, 2015.
This paper described the anatomy of the radial tunnel and the difficulty in accessing all portions of the tunnel from a single incision. The authors advocated multiple incisions for exposure of the entire tunnel.

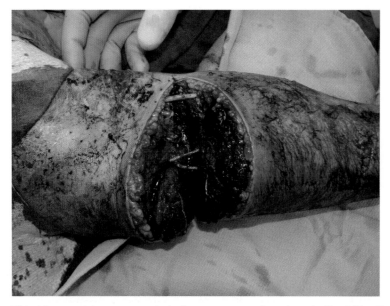

This 18-year-old man presents to the emergency department after falling through a glass door after a night of heavy drinking. He has a 17 cm laceration to his proximal forearm that penetrated deep to the fascia. On an examination, his vital signs are stable. His hand is perfused, and both the radial and the ulnar pulse are palpable. He is unable to antepose his thumb, and sensation is absent over the volar three and a half fingers and over the thenar eminence. He is able to flex the distal interphalangeal joints of all fingers and the proximal interphalangeal joints of his index and small fingers. His thumb interphalangeal flexion is intact. His flexor carpi ulnaris function is intact; however, the palmaris longus and the flexor carpi ulnaris tendons are not palpable and cannot be seen to contract. His ulnar nerve motor and sensory function in the hand is intact.

Description of the Problem

The direction of penetration of glass or other sharp objects into the forearm cannot be presumed to have occurred at right angles to the skin. Therefore all structures that traverse the forearm in the region of the laceration and proximal and distal to the laceration have to be assessed directly. Sensory and mixed motor-sensory nerves, arteries, muscles, and muscle tendon units all must be examined separately.

Key Anatomy

The cross-sectional anatomy of the forearm should be appreciated at the level of the injury. Based on a physical examination, surrounding structures adjacent to injured structures should be explored directly to assess for partial transections of tendons and muscle bellies. The surgical tactic depends on the physical examination findings in awake, sober patients. In patients who are not awake and sober, the exploration of the wound should progress in a logical fashion, either from superficial to deep or in another sequence that is specific to the surgeon (for example, arteries, nerves, and tendons).

Workup

PA and lateral radiographs are obtained to assess for fractures and retained foreign bodies such as glass.

Treatment

The treatment consists of surgical exploration and repair of injured structures. A prophylactic fasciotomy of the hand and forearm should be considered if the arterial supply to the hand has been disrupted for longer than 6 hours.

Alternatives

In an awake and sober patient with an entirely normal physical examination, the wound can be explored for retained glass. However, the wound can be closed primarily without a formal surgical exploration if the likelihood of glass being present is minimal.

Principles and Clinical Pearls

- The surgical tactic is usually based on the clinical examination, especially for cooperative patients.
- Surgeons should list the names of the injured surgical structures on the surgical drape before extending the incision proximally and distally. This will be a reminder to dissect and explore all structures whose normal continuity could not be confirmed on examination.
- Difficulties often arise in determining which tendon stumps proximally should be repaired to which tendon stumps distally. An evaluation of the tendons' relations to surrounding structures, including the overlying fascia, can assist the surgeon in this regard.

Pitfalls

Motor nerve connections in the forearm can give the impression of neural continuity even if a complete nerve laceration has occurred. For example, in a median to ulnar motor interconnection in the forearm, a complete median nerve laceration at the wrist might not affect the patient's thenar function adversely. Similarly, a median to ulnar motor interconnection in the forearm might prevent intrinsic muscle dysfunction in the presence of an ulnar nerve laceration in the proximal forearm or in the cubital tunnel.

Classic Reference

Leibovic SJ, Hastings H II. Martin-Gruber revisited. J Hand Surg Am 17:47, 1992.
This was an excellent discussion of the Martin-Gruber interconnections and how they can confuse the clinical examination of patients with nerve injuries in the volar forearm.

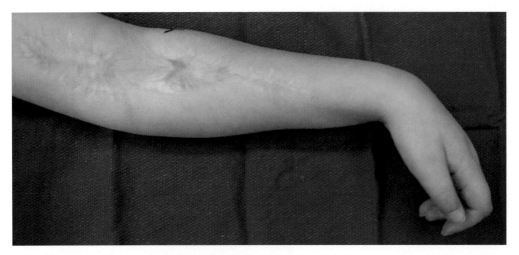

This 12-year-old girl had a laceration to her left volar forearm and a radial nerve injury. She presents 2 years after the injury and is unable to actively extend her wrist and fingers.

Description of the Problem

The girl has evidence of radial nerve palsy. She is unable to extend her wrist, thumb, and fingers. After 2 years, it is highly unlikely that a nerve repair will be successful.

Key Anatomy

The radial nerve innervates the extensor muscles of the wrist, thumb, and fingers. Direct branches from the radial nerve innervate the brachioradialis and the extensor carpi radialis longus muscles. The rest of the extensor muscles are innervated by the posterior interosseous nerve, a branch of the radial nerve. The order of innervation from proximal to distal is the following: the extensor carpi radialis brevis, the supinator, the extensor digitorum communis, the extensor digiti minimi, the extensor carpi ulnaris, the abductor pollicis longus, the extensor pollicis brevis, the extensor pollicis longus, and the extensor indicis proprius. This sequence is important in cases of radial nerve injury when reinnervation is progressing and may be predictably followed. For example, after neurapraxia of the radial nerve, a surgeon can reassure the patient that wrist extension will be the first function to return, followed by finger extension, and finally thumb extension.

Workup

The history of this injury should be carefully reviewed. Because the initial injury occurred 2 years ago, it is unlikely that a nerve repair or nerve grafting could be performed successfully. The possible donor muscles on the flexor side should be carefully evaluated. Good passive extension of the wrist and fingers is critical. PA and lateral radiographs are useful to ensure arthritis and old fractures are not present.

Treatment

Restoring wrist and finger extension is essential and will allow the patient to open her hand in space. Several options for tendon transfer are available; however, the standard transfer is the pronator teres muscle to the extensor carpi radialis brevis muscle, the palmaris longus tendon to the extensor pollicis longus tendon, and the flexor carpi ulnaris tendon to the extensor digitorum communis tendons. The surgery begins with isolation of the pronator teres muscle-tendon unit. It is important to take a long slip of periosteum of the pronator teres as it inserts onto the radius, because the pronator teres muscle-tendon unit is short, and all possible length is needed to be able to transfer it to the extensor carpi radialis brevis tendon. The proximal portion of the pronator teres muscle is dissected to allow free excursion of the muscle. This is woven into the side of the extensor carpi radialis brevis muscle. Through an ulnar excision, the flexor carpi ulnaris tendon is transected distally and proximally. The extensor digitorum communis tendons are found on the dorsum of the distal forearm and are sewn together to ensure a consistent cascade of all four fingers. The flexor carpi ulnaris tendon is then transferred onto the dorsum and sutured just proximal to this tendon coaptation. The palmaris longus tendon is found distally at the level of the wrist and is transferred to the extensor pollicis longus tendon in a similar fashion. A volar splint is placed, and the hand is immobilized for 3 weeks before active motion is initiated.

Alternatives

The best treatment for a radial nerve laceration is early, direct repair and/or grafting. Some recent data show the efficacy of nerve transfers from the median nerve to the radial nerve. However, most surgeons would choose to perform radial nerve tendon transfers, because they are easy and have a predictable outcome. An ongoing debate exists regarding the use of the flexor carpi radialis muscle-tendon unit as the motor for the extensor digitorum communis tendons instead of using the flexor carpi ulnaris muscle. Although many alternative tendon transfers have been proposed, those discussed previously seem to be the most straightforward.

Principles and Clinical Pearls

- The radial nerve tendon transfers are the most predictable tendon transfers for upper extremity nerve injuries.
- Suturing the extensor digitorum communis tendons will assist in proper tensioning of the finger extension tendon transfers.
- Retraining for this specific tendon transfer is fairly easy.

Pitfalls

The most common pitfalls result from improper tension on the tendon transfers. If the hand is not immobilized, some of the tendon transfers may pull through, necessitating retensioning of the tendon transfers. Some patients in whom the flexor carpi ulnaris tendon is harvested for finger extension may note weakness of grip and ulnar deviation.

Classic References

Bishop J, Ring D. Management of radial nerve palsy associated with humeral shaft fracture: a decision analysis model. J Hand Surg Am 34:991, 2009.
Many cases of radial nerve palsy are related to humeral shaft fractures. This was an excellent study discussing observation versus early exploration of the radial nerve.

Sammer DM, Chung KC. Tendon transfers: part I. Principles of transfer and transfers for radial nerve palsy. Plast Reconstr Surg 123:169, 2009.
The principles of tendon transfer for radial nerve palsy were discussed, along with the authors' recommendations for optimal tendon transfers.

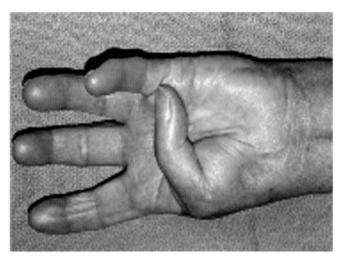

This 57-year-old man presents to his primary care doctor because he is unable to use his left hand. He cannot feel the tips of his thumb and index fingers and has difficulty buttoning his shirt and gripping larger objects such as bottles and cans of food or beer. On an examination, sensation is absent over the median nerve distribution, and his thenar musculature has severe wasting. He has full-strength, active flexion of the interphalangeal joint of his thumb and of the distal interphalangeal joint of his index finger.

Description of the Problem

Chronic carpal tunnel syndrome is a cause of low median nerve palsy. Compression of the median nerve proximally in the forearm, with a resultant complete palsy, leads to a concurrent anterior interosseous nerve palsy (an inability to flex the distal interphalangeal joints of the index and possibly the middle finger and the interphalangeal joint of the thumb). The hallmarks of low median nerve palsy are an inability to antepose the thumb and altered sensation over the volar aspect of the thumb, index, middle, and ring fingers.

Key Anatomy

The median nerve passes deep to the superficial head of the pronator teres in the proximal forearm and travels distally in the forearm deep to the flexor digitorum superficialis muscle. The palmar cutaneous branch of the median nerve exits the median nerve approximately 5 cm proximal to the wrist crease, and this branch enters the hand immediately ulnar to the flexor carpi radialis muscle. Numbness over the thenar eminence suggests proximal median nerve entrapment or injury. The median nerve extends to the distal forearm from under the flexor digitorum superficialis tendon of the middle finger and enters the carpal tunnel in its superficial radial aspect. The median nerve motor branch innervates the opponens pollicis and the abductor pollicis brevis muscles and the superficial head of the flexor pollicis brevis muscle. Common digital nerve branches travel beneath the superficial palmar arterial arch and innervate the skin overlying the volar aspect of the thumb, index, and middle fingers and the radial half of the ring finger.

Workup

Electrophysiologic assessment by nerve conduction velocity and electromyography are performed to document axonal loss and to localize the lesion. Plain radiographs are obtained if a mass is suspected or with a history of trauma, and an MRI is obtained if a soft tissue mass or a synovial compression is suspected.

Treatment

Median nerve decompression can arrest the progression of the axon loss and might restore some sensation. It rarely leads to motor recovery. Treatment for a high median nerve palsy includes a tendon transfer of the brachioradialis to the flexor pollicis longus and a side-to-side transfer of the flexor digitorum profundus tendons of the index and middle fingers to the ring finger. If high median nerve function is normal in low median nerve palsy, a tendon transfer may improve thumb anteposition. Multiple donors have been described; the choice is based on the surgeon's preference and the availability of donors. The flexor digitorum superficialis tendon to the third or fourth finger can be rerouted around the flexor carpi ulnaris muscle or the palmar fascia for a strong, active opponensplasty. Other possible donor muscle-tendon units include the extensor indicis proprius rerouted around the ulna, the abductor digiti minimi routed across the palm, and the palmaris longus elongated with volar fascia. All transfers are fixed to the tendon of the abductor pollicis brevis and are immobilized postoperatively for 3 weeks. Hand therapy is then initiated to instruct the patient in the use of the transfer.

Alternatives

Patients who have no appreciable disability do not need a surgical transfer of tendons to restore function. Other differential diagnostic possibilities include a C6 or C8 radiculopathy, anterior interosseous nerve palsy, Parsonage-Turner syndrome, and other proximal nerve entrapments. Peripheral neuropathies such as Guillain-Barré or Charcot-Marie-Tooth have been described. Leprosy may lead to both motor and sensory palsies of the peripheral nerves.

Principles and Clinical Pearls

- Thumb anteposition or opposition can be restored by a number of tendon transfers. No one transfer is favored, because they all have the same function—positioning the thumb to do work. Abductorplasty is not a "strength" transfer per se, but rather a transfer that places the thumb in a suitable position for both pinching and grasping large objects. This patient underwent a transfer of the palmaris longus tendon and elongation by the palmar fascia (a Camitz transfer).
- Anterior interosseous nerve palsies should be differentiated from proximal median nerve compressions. The main differentiating feature is that anterior interosseous nerve palsies are motor palsies, and proximal median nerve palsies include sensory loss in the fingers and the palm.

Pitfalls

In general, tendon transfers should be sutured more tightly so that some stretch can be expected after immobilization is discontinued and use of the transfer begins. For all tendon transfers, the principles of a stable soft tissue bed and one tendon–one function should be followed. Thumb web space adduction contractures should be treated (either by therapy or surgical release) before a tendon transfer is performed.

Classic Reference

Cooney WP. Tendon transfer for median nerve palsy. Hand Clin 4:155, 1988.
The author provided a good review of available transfers for restoring hand function after high and low median nerve palsy.

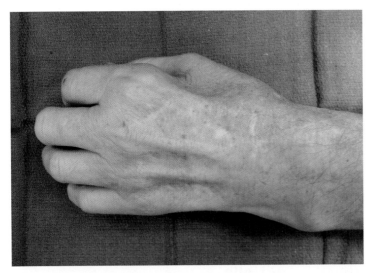

This 41-year-old man presents to his primary care doctor because he is unable to hold a key and his hand feels "sloppy" and weak. He had noticed a hollow space between his thumb and index finger metacarpals on the back of his hand and a prominence of the extensor tendons over the dorsum of his hand. He reported that his small finger "stuck out" from the rest of his hand, and that when attempting to grasp a large object, his small and ring fingers tended to push the object out of his palm rather than encircle it. On an examination, he had substantially decreased sensation over the ulnar aspect of his small finger and the ulnar aspect of his ring finger volarly and dorsally, and he had normal sensation over the dorsal ulnar aspect of his hand and palm. He could not adduct his small finger to his ring finger and could not easily flex the metacarpophalangeal joints of his small and ring fingers. When the metacarpophalangeal joints were blocked from hyperextending, the interphalangeal joints of his ring and small fingers extended fully (a Bouvier test, indicating an intact central slip and a triangular ligament).

Description of the Problem

Low ulnar nerve palsy results in substantial loss of the motor function of the hand, including the loss of side pinch and of the ability to abduct and adduct the fingers, with clawing of the ring and small fingers. The ulnar one and a half fingers may have sensory loss if the lesion affecting the nerve includes motor and sensory fibers. High ulnar nerve palsies have paradoxically less clawing than lower palsies, because the flexor digitorum profundus tendons to the ring and small fingers are affected, and proximal interphalangeal and distal interphalangeal joint flexion is decreased as a result. Patients usually are concerned with inability to pinch, finger clawing, and the small finger abduction posture.

Key Anatomy

The ulnar nerve courses behind the medial epicondyle and enters the forearm between the two heads of the flexor carpi ulnaris. It travels distally superficial to the flexor digitorum muscle belly. The dorsal cutaneous branch of the ulnar nerve exits the main body of the nerve approximately 5 cm proximal to the ulnar styloid. The branch courses distally and crosses to the dorsum of the hand, approximately 2 cm distal to the ulnar styloid. It can usually be palpated directly over the triquetrum in this location. The ulnar nerve enters the hand deep to the volar carpal ligament (which forms the roof of the Guyon canal) ulnar and deep to the ulnar artery. Three branches exist: the motor branch to the hypothenar muscles, the sensory branch to the palmar aspect of the ulnar one and a half digits, and the deep motor branch to the volar and dorsal interosseous muscles, the ulnar two lumbricals, the adductor pollicis, and the deep head of the flexor pollicis brevis muscle. The motor branch leaves the main trunk of the ulnar nerve on its deep ulnar aspect and dives into the floor of the hand deep to the fibrous leading edge of the flexor digiti minimi muscle. It innervates the muscles listed previously. The final muscle innervated by the deep branch of the ulnar nerve is the first dorsal interosseous muscle.

Workup

Electrophysiologic assessment by nerve conduction velocity and electromyography are performed to document axonal loss and to localize the lesion proximodistally. The distal ulnar tunnel has three zones. From proximal to distal, these zones are motor and sensory, motor only, and sensory only in zones 1, 2, and 3, respectively. Plain radiographs and CT scans can be used to assess for hook of hamate fractures, and MRI can be used to assess for soft tissue lesions. If ulnar artery thrombosis is suspected, then an angiogram can assist in the diagnosis. Maintenance of metacarpophalangeal, proximal interphalangeal, and distal interphalangeal joint motion and soft tissue compliance is necessary if tendon transfer is to be performed. Hand therapy should minimize or eliminate joint contractures, and the soft tissues through which the transfers are to be placed should be soft and well vascularized.

Treatment

The preferred method to minimize a Froment sign and strengthen side pinch is transfer of the extensor carpi radialis longus or the extensor carpi radialis brevis (elongated with palmaris longus) around the intermetacarpal space ulnar to the index metacarpal and insertion into the adductor aponeurosis at the ulnar aspect of the thumb metacarpophalangeal joint. The extensor digiti minimi can be rerouted to correct the fixed abduction of the small finger (a Wartenberg sign), and similar rerouting of the extensor indicis proprius can assist in index finger abduction and stabilization of the index finger with side pinch.

Transfer of the flexor digitorum superficialis tendons of the middle and ring fingers through the lumbrical canals to the ulnolateral bands of the index, middle, and ring fingers and the radiolateral band of the small finger can be performed. A four-tailed palmaris longus graft can be transferred to the extensor carpi radialis longus or the extensor carpi radialis brevis tendon and the grafts rerouted through the lumbrical canals. The transfer is inserted into the lateral band or into the volar aspect of the base of the proximal phalanx to rebalance the hand and assist in metacarpophalangeal joint flexion with either flexor digitorum superficialis activity or with wrist extension activity (synergistic finger flexion).

Alternatives

Splints to immobilize the interphalangeal joint of the thumb or arthrodesis of the interphalangeal joint of the thumb can prevent interphalangeal joint flexion with attempted side pinch (a Froment sign.) Hand-based splints to maintain neutral or slight flexion of the metacarpophalangeal joints while at rest and to block their hyperextension during attempted digital extension can serve as anticlaw devices. Hyperextended metacarpophalangeal joints can also be treated by volar plate capsulodesis through a volar approach and incision of the A1 pulley, followed by volar plate advancement.

Principles and Clinical Pearls

- Tendon transfer to rebalance the hand following low ulnar nerve palsy should strengthen lateral pinch and eliminate clawing.
- The treatment of high ulnar nerve palsies should not include transfer of the flexor digitorum profundus tendons to those of the index and middle fingers, because the claw deformity will increase after the transfer.
- In general, tendon transfers for ulnar nerve palsy can insert into the lateral bands (if a Bouvier test has demonstrated an intact central slip and triangular ligament structure and function) or into the base of the proximal phalanges (if a Bouvier test indicates extensor mechanism function incompetence or if additional grip power is required for the patient's work).

Pitfalls

Injudicious handling of the tendons during a transfer can cause focal adhesions to develop and require later tenolysis to restore glide and pullthrough. After a microneurorrhaphy of a high ulnar nerve laceration, clawing will worsen initially as the nerve reinnervates the flexor digitorum muscle-tendon units and will subside only when the intrinsic muscles of the hand are reinnervated.

Classic Reference

Fischer T, Nagy L, Buechler U. Restoration of pinch grip in ulnar nerve paralysis: extensor carpi radialis longus to adductor pollicis and abductor pollicis longus to first dorsal interosseous tendon transfers. J Hand Surg Br 28:28, 2003.

This clinical review provided technical pointers on how to improve index finger abduction and strengthen thumb pinch after ulnar nerve palsy, resulting in a more stable, strong side pinch.

76 High Median and Ulnar Nerve Palsy

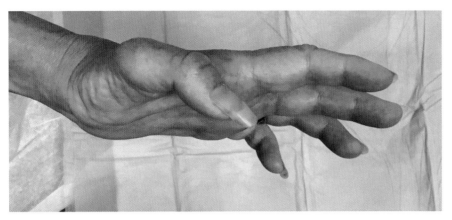

This 63-year-old woman presents to her primary care doctor with a history of progressive weakness and deformity of both hands. She has a history of insulin dependent diabetes mellitus and had been told that she had a neuropathy. On an examination, she has flattening of her volar arch, wasting of both thenar and hypothenar eminences, clawing of her fingers, and an inability to pinch. Sensation is decreased over the volar surface of her hand. She cannot grasp large objects, because she is unable to initiate flexion. (Photo courtesy of Charles Goldfarb, MD.)

Description of the Problem

Combined high median nerve and ulnar nerve palsy is severely detrimental to hand function, because all intrinsic hand muscles, extrinsic digital flexors, and volar sensation are affected. The only functional muscle-tendon units available for transfer are those supplied by the radial nerve and the posterior interosseous nerve (the brachioradialis [BR], the extensor carpi radialis longus [ECRL], the extensor carpi radialis longus [ECRL], the extensor carpi radialis brevis [ECRB], the extensor digiti communis [EDC], the extensor indicis proprius [EIP], the extensor digiti quinti [EDQ], the extensor carpi ulnaris [ECU], the abductor pollicis longus [AbPL], the extensor pollicis longus [EPL], and the extensor pollicis brevis [EPB]).

Key Anatomy

Patients with combined high median and ulnar nerve palsy are unable to antepose the thumb because of the loss of thenar muscle function (primarily the median nerve) and are unable to pinch because of loss of adductor pollicis function (the ulnar nerve) and flexor pollicis longus (FPL) function (the anterior interosseous branch of the median nerve). The loss of lumbrical function and interosseous function results in metacarpophalangeal (MCP) joint hyperextension because of unopposed pull of the long digital extensors. The small finger is held in abduction (a Wartenberg sign) because of unopposed pull of the EDQ. (The vector of the EDQ as it crosses the MCP joint dorsally tends to result in MCP abduction.)

Workup

A neurologic assessment is performed to identify correctable causes of peripheral neuropathies. More frequently encountered causes include diabetes mellitus, vitamin B_{12} deficiency, hypothyroidism, rheumatoid disease, and systemic lupus erythematosus. Plain radiographs and MRI of the cervical spine can help to rule out nerve root pathology. Family members are evaluated to assess for familial polyneuropathies. The patient's feet are examined to assess for systemic neuropathies.

Treatment

The underlying condition causing the neuropathic changes in the hands is diagnosed first. If necessary, neurologic and medical consultations are sought. If tendon transfers will be performed, all joints across which transfers are to be rerouted should be soft and fully mobile, and the soft tissues should be compliant and well vascularized. Available donors include the brachioradialis, one of the radial wrist extensors, the EIP, the EDQ, and the AbPL. Pinch can be strengthened by transfer of a radial wrist extensor elongated with palmaris longus tendon to the insertion of the adductor pollicis. Thumb interphalangeal joint flexion can be strengthened by transfer of the brachioradialis to the FPL tendon. Finger flexion can be restored by transfer of a radial wrist extensor to the FDP tendons, and MCP joint hyperextension should be corrected by capsulodesis of the volar MCP joints (the volar plate.) Thumb abduction can be achieved by transfer of the EIP around the ulnar aspect of the forearm to the tendon of the AbPB.

Alternatives

Alternative treatments include arthrodesis and tenodesis of the paralyzed joints. If the BR is needed elsewhere or is deemed inadequate for transfer, fusion of the thumb interphalangeal joint or tenodesis across the joint can be performed. Similarly, FDP tenodesis to the distal radius is an option instead of direct transfer of a wrist extensor. Omer has also suggested index ray amputation and a radiodorsal skin flap transposed volarly to restore some sensation to the palm.

Principles and Clinical Pearls

- The principles of tendon transfers must be adhered to in patients with high median and ulnar nerve palsy, given the paucity of donor muscle-tendon units.
- An evaluation for reversible causes of peripheral polyneuropathy is essential, including those testable serologically and those caused by peripheral nerve compression or nerve root compression in the lower cervical spinal cord.
- Tendon transfer procedures should be staged to facilitate relearning the transfers' functions in an organized fashion to maximize outcome.
- Sensory restoration is difficult, particularly by a pedicled transposition of radial nerve–innervated tissue to the palm.

Pitfalls

Planning of the transfers based on the tissues available and planning of the postoperative therapy should be carried out in an organized fashion before the first transfer. Tendon transfers are not performed in patients with a progressive polyneuropathy; splinting alone (either static or dynamic) is best used to maximize function. Sensory dysfunction will compromise the function of the most technically well done transfer because of the lack of appropriate feedback.

Classic Reference

Omer GE Jr. Reconstruction of the forearm and hand after peripheral nerve injuries. In Omer GE Jr, Spinner M, Van Beek AL, eds. Management of Peripheral Nerve Problems, ed 2. Philadelphia: WB Saunders, 1998. *This chapter described the various considerations inherent in the transfer of any muscle-tendon unit after a peripheral nerve injury of the upper extremity. The authors stressed careful planning of the entire cascade of procedures to be performed.*

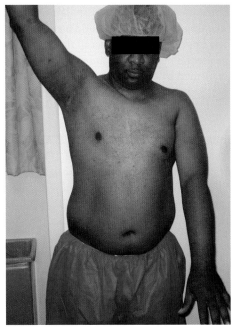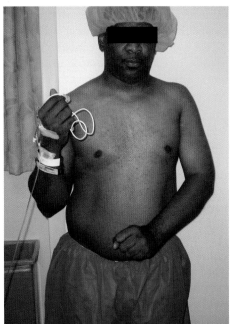

This 37-year-old construction worker presents to the emergency department after a work-related injury in which a 75-pound box fell from a height of 20 feet directly onto his left shoulder and neck. He was unable to move his arm initially; however, after transport to the emergency department, he begins to feel electrical sensations emanating from his neck down to his anterior arm, past his elbow and to his thumb. He has a large hematoma at the base of his neck and is tender to palpation over his entire shoulder girdle. A physical examination reveals absent sensation over the deltoid muscle and over the lateral aspect of his forearm. He is unable to contract his deltoid and biceps brachii muscles, and his wrist extension is extremely weak. He has intact elbow extension, wrist flexion, and finger flexion and extension and normal intrinsic hand function. He has intact sensation over the medial arm and forearm and over the ulnar side of his hand and wrist. Pupils are equal and reactive to light. Radial and ulnar pulses are palpable and fully intact.

Description of the Problem

Brachial plexus lesions in adults can be grouped into four main types: upper plexus, lower plexus, complete, and mixed. The upper plexus lesions, such as this patient has, involve injuries to the C5 and the C6 nerve roots. They include combined injuries to the axillary and musculocutaneous nerves. The lower plexus injuries typically involve injury to the C8 and T1 roots (sometimes C7) and resemble a combined median and ulnar nerve injury. Complete brachial plexus palsies affect the entire plexus and result in a paralyzed, anesthetic arm. Mixed, or partial, palsies present with several independent sites of nerve dysfunction that cannot be attributed to a solitary lesion. A full motor and sensory examination, including the periscapular musculature, should be performed. Upper extremity perfusion is assessed if scapulothoracic dissociation is suspected.

Key Anatomy

The anatomy of the brachial plexus is well known. It originates as nerve roots C5, C6, C7, C8, and T1 (presuming the plexus is in the normal location, that is, not prefixed or postfixed). The roots combine to form the upper, middle, and lower trunks. The trunks divide (the divisions) to form the medial, lateral, and posterior cords. The lateral cord terminates as the musculocutaneous nerve. Medial and lateral cords send fibers to form the median nerve. The medial cord terminates as the ulnar nerve. The posterior cord is formed by fibers from the upper, middle, and lower trunks and terminates as the radial nerve and the axillary nerve. The dorsal scapular nerve emanates from the C5 root, and the suprascapular nerve is a branch of the upper trunk. Lateral and medial pectoral nerves are branches of the lateral and medial cords, respectively. The upper and lower subscapular nerves are branches off of the posterior cord (as is the thoracodorsal nerve.) The medial brachial and antebrachial cutaneous nerves are branches of the medial cord. The long thoracic nerve is formed from the C5, C6, and C7 roots.

Workup

CT myelography or MRI of the cervical spine is performed to assess for nerve root avulsion (as evidenced by the presence of pseudomeningoceles and a sensory nerve action potential from an anesthetic dermatome). If they are avulsed, then the injury may be considered permanent. If the nerve roots or the brachial plexus has been lacerated, stretched, or avulsed, then the sensory nerve action potentials would be absent, thus indicating a postganglionic injury (and not an avulsion of the nerve roots themselves.)

Treatment

In penetrating injuries of the brachial plexus, exploration of the supraclavicular plexus (posterior to the anterior scalene muscle in the neck) and the infraclavicular plexus (deep to the pectoralis minor and medial to the coracoid process of the scapula) can proceed, with the goal of nerve repair. If nerve repair is either not possible or unsuccessful, then tendon transfers, nerve transfers, or free-functioning muscle transfers can be performed to restore some upper extremity function. Several reliable nerve transfers that have been used to restore shoulder abduction are a spinal accessory nerve transfer to the suprascapular nerve and a radial nerve branch to the deep head of the triceps transfer to the posterior axillary nerve. Transfers to restore elbow flexion include an ulnar nerve fascicle to the biceps brachii branch of the musculocutaneous nerve or a bifascicular transfer involving an ulnar nerve to the biceps branch transfer combined with a median nerve to the brachialis branch transfer. Sensory nerve transfers and those such as an anterior interosseous nerve transfer to the deep branch of the ulnar nerve are considered somewhat experimental, and the results of these transfers are the topic of lively debate.

Alternatives

In a complete brachial plexus injury, shoulder arthrodesis (if trapezius muscle function is acceptable) can be performed, along with a transhumeral amputation, followed by fitting of an assistive prosthesis.

Principles and Clinical Pearls

- Nonemergent treatment can be performed, unless a vascular injury is present after a penetrating or nonpenetrating trauma.
- The presence of Horner syndrome indicates lower plexus root avulsions and a poor prognosis.
- If intraplexal dissection is to be performed after repair of a vascular injury, a vascular surgeon should be present for the approach and prepared for vascular bypass or reconstruction.
- The most reliable nerve transfers are those that restore elbow flexion and shoulder abduction within the first 12 months of injury.

Pitfalls

These surgical cases should be attempted only in centers with expertise in the area. Knowledge of the anatomy of the brachial plexus and of the exact location or locations of the neural injuries is necessary before attempting any surgical treatment, either intraplexal or extraplexal.

Classic Reference

Shin AY, Spinner RJ, Steinmann SP, Bishop AT. Adult traumatic brachial plexus injuries. J Am Acad Orthop Surg 13:382, 2005.
This excellent review article discussed the relevant considerations guiding treatment of adults with brachial plexus injuries.

78 Gunshot Wound to the Axilla

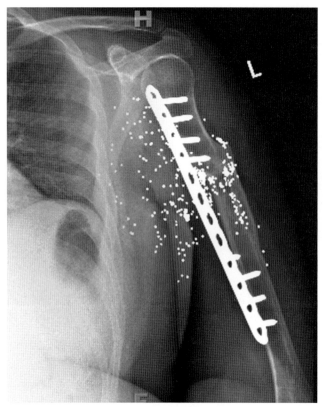

This 32-year-old man presents to the emergency department in shock from a self-inflicted gunshot wound to the axilla. He was attempting to commit suicide, but the gun slipped as it was being discharged, and the shot entered his anterior axilla. He was discovered by a family member, who applied pressure and called 911. The patient was transported to the emergency department. His hemodynamic status has been stabilized, and a physical examination of his arm reveals an open humeral shaft fracture, a large wound through his anterior axillary fold, and profuse bleeding from the wound. He has patchy sensory deficits in his entire arm, although his radial and ulnar pulses are both palpable. Elbow flexion and shoulder abduction cannot be assessed; however, he has active wrist and finger extension. The patient is not able to actively flex his fingers or abduct or adduct his fingers or thumb.

Description of the Problem

Missile wounds to the axilla present a mutilayered management dilemma for surgeons. First, the hemodynamic status must be stabilized, and concomitant injury to the chest or the great vessels needs to be ruled out. The vascular and neurologic (motor and sensory) status of the arm is examined, and the bony continuity is assessed with a physical examination and radiographs. Any bony injury is treated like an open fracture in patients with a large open shotgun wound, and operative irrigation and debridement are performed. Bony stability is achieved, and vascular injuries are either repaired or, more typically, bypassed. Because nerve injuries tend to not be neurotmetic in terms of their continuity, exploration early in the course of a patient's care is ill advised.

Key Anatomy

The subclavian artery and vein pass posterior to the clavicle and enter the arm deep to the pectoralis minor muscle between the medial, lateral, and posterior cords. The brachial plexus and the axillary artery and vein are contained within the axillary sheath.

Workup

Patients are evaluated for Horner syndrome. Angiography might be necessary in the acute phase if vascular injury is suspected or on a delayed basis if an arterial aneurysm or pseudoaneurysm is thought to have developed. Plain radiographs are obtained to evaluate the distribution of missiles and the location and the pattern of fractures. An electrophysiologic assessment is performed to localize diffuse lesions, and, along with repeated physical examinations, it allows a longitudinal evaluation of improvement.

Treatment

The initial treatment of these injuries is to restore hemodynamic stability. Compromised blood flow to the arm is restored by means of an arterial repair or bypass. The brachial plexus can be explored on a delayed basis if the treatment of one or more localized lesions can possibly restore function; for example, an isolated lesion of the posterior cord, leading to radial nerve and axillary nerve dysfunction. Alternatively, nerve transfers can be performed on a delayed basis. In this clinical situation, the surgeon needs to be certain that the nerves being transferred were not affected by the initial injury.

Alternatives

There are no treatment alternatives.

Principles and Clinical Pearls

- The brachial plexus lesions are the least of this patient's immediate problems.
- Intraplexal dissection requires caution, and the assistance of a vascular surgeon should be arranged preoperatively.
- The nerve injuries caused by shotgun wounds to the axilla rarely involve the loss of nerve continuity, and they can usually be followed over time for improvement or for an advancing Tinel sign in mixed motor and sensory nerves.

Pitfalls

Surgeons should resist the urge to explore penetrating injuries early unless the penetrating object was a knife. The best plan for patients with gunshot injuries to the brachial plexus is to observe and assess for recovery over time.

Classic Reference

Lin PH, Koffron AJ, Guske PJ, Lujan HJ, Heilizer TJ, Yario RF, Tatooles CJ. Penetrating injuries of the subclavian artery. Am J Surg 185:580, 2003.
Injury to the brachial plexus was the causative factor in patients' long-term morbidity after a gun or knife injury to the subclavian artery.

Soft Tissue Defects

79 Exposed Flexor Tendon

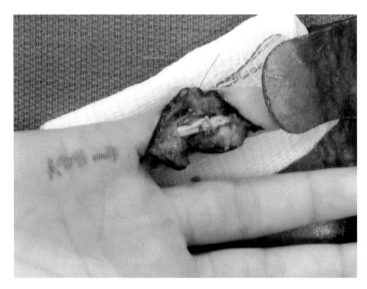

This patient has undergone a flexor tendon repair in zone 2 and has a large volar soft tissue defect exposing the tendon.

Description of the Problem

An exposed flexor tendon is a difficult wound problem, because the tendon will not take a skin graft. A fresh tendon repair needs good soft tissue coverage to allow postoperative therapy.

Key Anatomy

The flexor tendon is in a protected space within the flexor tendon sheath. This sheath provides a good covering to allow skin grafting. However, once the sheath is missing, the bare flexor tendon—even with its paratenon—has difficulty supporting a skin graft. The need for range of motion will preclude the use of direct skin grafting. A wide variety of flaps are available based on the detailed neurovascular anatomy of the hand.

Workup

The patient's wound is examined. If the flexor tendon repair is adequate, all attempts should be made to cover the wound primarily. In this finger, the scarred tissue will not allow direct closure. Therefore the surgeon needs to determine intraoperatively other possible areas for soft tissue. These include tissues in the finger itself, in the proximal hand, and on adjacent digits. Patients should be counseled preoperatively about the possibility of local flap coverage and skin grafting.

Treatment

The optimal flap in this case is a cross-finger flap from the ring finger. This is harvested by elevating the entire dorsum of the ring finger proximal phalanx skin based along the ulnar aspect of the ring finger. Cleland ligaments are released on that side to allow full freedom of the dorsal flap onto the volar surface of the small finger. The peritenon is carefully preserved on the dorsum of the ring finger, and full thickness is harvested from the antecubital fossa to fill this area. The fingers are kept together for 3 weeks postoperatively. After 10 days, when the dorsal skin graft is adherent, early active range of motion exercises can be initiated to help rehabilitate the flexor tendon repair. Three weeks postoperatively, the flap connection is separated, and the small wound is closed. Further range of motion therapy is based on the protocols for flexor tendon rehabilitation.

Alternatives

Many alternatives are available for flap coverage in the small finger, including homodigital island flaps and venous flow-through flaps. However, cross-finger flaps are the most straightforward and reliable for coverage.

Principles and Clinical Pearls

- The flexor tendon sheath provides a good layer of coverage for the flexor tendon. It should be preserved as well as possible in any flexor tendon procedure to allow skin grafting.
- Cross-finger flaps are a workhorse flap for the hand and should be an alternative for all surgeons.
- Surgeons should know the homodigital island flaps and venous flow-through flaps, because their use can prevent a secondary surgery.

Pitfalls

Pitfalls are related to chronic exposure of a flexor tendon. If a wound breaks down and the tendon becomes exposed, it will rupture and lead to extensive, significant problems requiring staged tendon reconstruction.

Classic References

Garlick JW, Goodwin A, Wolter K, Agarwal JP. Arterialized venous flow-through flaps in the reconstruction of digital defects: case series and review of the literature. Hand (N Y) 10:184, 2015.
Venous flow-through flaps were reviewed. This is an excellent technique that allows microsurgical reconstruction using an artery to the flap and an artery leaving the flap. It is both a vein graft and a soft tissue flap.

Katz R. The anterograde homodigital neurovascular island flap. J Hand Surg Am 38:1226, 2013.
Homodigital island flaps have a large role in finger reconstruction; however, they require sacrificing a digital nerve. They are useful in areas needing large resurfacing with sensate glabrous skin.

Rehim S, Chung K. Local flaps of the hand. Hand Clin 30:137, 2014.
This was an excellent overall review of local flaps of the hand, including cross-finger flaps.

Tendon: Atraumatic Conditions (Tenosynovitis)

80 Trigger Finger

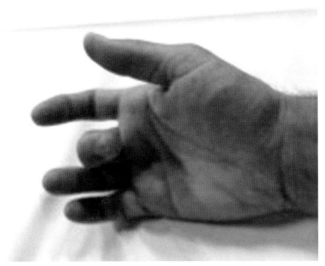

This 48-year-old insulin-dependent diabetic presents with a 6-week history of painful clicking and locking of his right middle finger. He reports no antecedent trauma. His HgbA1c levels have been steady between 6.0% and 7.0%. The pain and locking are the worst in the morning. Occasionally, he has to extend his finger passively to alleviate the flexed position. A physical examination reveals tenderness over the A1 pulley of the middle finger. The proximal interphalangeal joint cannot be extended passively past 20 degrees of flexion. A small, tender 2 mm immobile round mass is present at the metacarpophalangeal (MCP) flexion crease of the finger, distal to the point of maximal tenderness.

Description of the Problem

Triggering of the finger or the thumb occurs because of a size mismatch between the A1 pulley and the tendons gliding beneath it. It can be associated with subtle digital swelling or a proximal interphalangeal joint flexion deformity, along with a volar retinacular ganglion cyst (a ganglion cyst of the flexor tendon sheath.) Although locking is not always present, tenderness at the A1 pulley is essentially pathognomonic for this condition. This patient has a trigger finger, with a volar retinacular ganglion cyst of the flexor sheath. The differential diagnosis includes a giant cell tumor of the tendon sheath, an epidermal inclusion cyst, a neurofibroma, a schwannoma (see Chapter 98), a hemangioma (see Chapter 95), an arteriovenous malformation, MCP joint osteoarthritis (see Chapter 11), and MCP joint inflammatory arthritis (see Chapter 14).

Key Anatomy

The thumb A1 pulley is immediately subjacent to the radial digital nerve (RDN) of the thumb, which lies less than 2 mm deep to the skin and is in danger of injury during a surgical approach. The radial digital nerve of the index finger and the radially situated lumbrical to the index finger lie radial to the A1 pulley of the index finger. The A1 pulley inserts and originates from the volar plate of the MCP joint. It can be divided without loss of active digital range of motion.

Workup

If the origin of the small mass is not known, an ultrasound may be obtained. If MCP osteoarthritis is suspected, a PA plain radiograph of the hand is obtained. Trigger finger can co-exist with MCP joint osteoarthritis.

Treatment

Splinting of the MCP and the PIP joints at night is frequently ineffective. Long-term blood glucose control should be sought in diabetics. A mixture of corticosteroids either with or without local anesthetics can be directly injected into the sheath and/or surrounding the flexor sheath. Injections can be repeated as necessary, although data show a transient rise in blood glucose levels for 2 days, followed by a reliable return to baseline. Pain at the injection site is common. Operative treatment consists of direct release of the A1 pulley. If the thumb is operated on, then the radial digital nerve should be identified and retracted radially (away from the sheath.) After the release, either active or passive digital motion is performed to confirm the absence of locking or triggering. The volar retinacular cyst is excised.

Alternatives

After severe trauma, a saddle syndrome (lumbrical-interosseous adhesion syndrome) should be considered. Symptomatic MCP joint osteoarthritis should be ruled out before a pulley release.

Principles and Clinical Pearls

- A volar aponeurosis pulley proximal to the A1 pulley may result in persistent triggering after A1 release. It should be released surgically.
- The radial digital nerve of the thumb and index finger should be isolated for a trigger release of these digits.
- Fixed proximal interphalangeal flexion contracture persists even after a surgical pulley release and after corticosteroid injections.

Pitfalls

Complications of treatment include a digital nerve injury, wound dehiscence, an infection (of the wound or the flexor sheath), stiffness, pain, and, rarely, recurrence.

Classic Reference

Carrozzella J, Stern PJ, Von Kuster LC. Transection of radial digital nerve of the thumb during trigger release. J Hand Surg Am 14:198, 1989.
This article highlighted the position of the thumb radial digital nerve at risk.

81 de Quervain Tenosynovitis

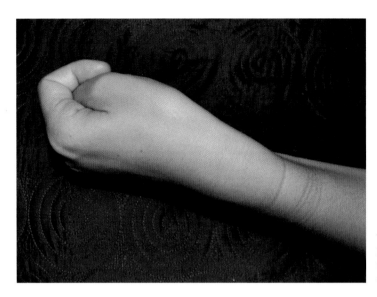

This woman has a history of wrist pain with lifting her baby. On an examination, she has marked radial-sided pain with forced ulnar deviation of the wrist.

Description of the Problem

de Quervain tenosynovitis is a condition in which the first dorsal extensor compartment tendons—the abductor pollicis longus (APL) and the extensor pollicis brevis (EPB)—are inflamed as they run through the tight extensor compartment. This is common in young mothers who lift their babies for feeding or diaper changing.

Key Anatomy

Several unique features of the local anatomy (one each for the APL tendons and the EPB tendon) are responsible for the pathophysiology and the complications. The extensor retinaculum is normally very tight. Any swelling of these tendons will cause pain and discomfort. This first compartment is probably divided into two subcompartments (one each for the APL and EPB tendons) by a septum. Steroid injections may not be effective if only one subcompartment is infiltrated. Furthermore, 90% of patients have two or more slips of the APL tendon. When the first dorsal compartment is released, it is necessary to confirm that both the APL and the EPB are free and not just the multiple slips of the APL in one subcompartment. Finally, the radial sensory nerve branches are at great risk in surgery, because they run directly over the extensor retinaculum.

Workup

Patients will present to clinic with severe radial-sided wrist pain. Common inciting activities include nursing babies or strenuous hammering from new home projects. With a careful history-taking, patients may reveal a new event that is temporally related to the pain. Differential diagnoses that should be ruled out include thumb carpometacarpal joint arthritis, scaphoid problems, and, rarely, intersection syndrome. The Finkelstein test, in which the thumb is grasped by the examiner and the wrist is passively ulnarly deviated, will almost always cause tenderness along the extensor tendons just proximal to the radial styloid. This test is pathognomonic for de Quervain tenosynovitis.

Treatment

The initial treatment for de Quervain tenosynovitis is a steroid injection into the first dorsal compartment. Patients should be informed that mild atrophy and/or skin discoloration can develop from this superficial injection. Up to two injections 6 weeks apart may be given. Some hand surgeons prescribe a long opponens splint, but these are poorly tolerated, and studies have shown variable efficacy. Altering the behavior, that is, changing diapers with the baby on the floor rather than lifting the body onto a changing table, may decrease the pain symptoms. Usually, young mothers will no longer have this problem as their child grows older; therefore surgery is not needed.

Surgery is recommended only after at least two steroid injections have been given and after the inciting activity has been discontinued for some time. A small transverse incision is made along the radial wrist, approximately 1 cm proximal to the radial styloid. The radial sensory nerve branches are identified and gently retracted. The extensor retinaculum of the first dorsal compartment is opened as dorsally as possible to create a ledge that will minimize volar subluxation of the tendons. Surgeons should look for a septum separating any subcompartments; this should be released. The tendons are retracted to clearly identify the EPB (and its distal muscle belly) versus the multiple slips of the APL. Overrelease of the extensor retinaculum is avoided to minimize subluxation of the tendons.

Alternatives

A steroid injection is the first line of treatment. Iontophoresis and therapy may be prescribed for patients who do not want an injection; however, the results are variable. In many patients, de Quervain tenosynovitis is a self-limited problem. Surgery is reserved for severe, unremitting cases.

Principles and Clinical Pearls

- de Quervain tenosynovitis is usually cured with steroid injections and activity modification.
- The particular anatomy, as discussed previously, determines the pathophysiology and complications.
- Three major complications can be prevented: sensory nerve injury, incomplete release, and overrelease.

Pitfalls

A sensory nerve injury may lead to extreme neuroma pain. Iatrogenic injuries should be repaired intraoperatively. The first dorsal compartment can be incompletely released if careful inspection for a dorsal subcompartment containing the EPB tendon is not performed; continued pain will result. Last, extended release of the extensor retinaculum with release of the proximal and distal fascia may lead to volar subluxation of the extensor tendons during active flexion of the wrist.

Classic References

Ilyas AM. Nonsurgical treatment for de Quervain's tenosynovitis. J Hand Surg Am 34:928, 2009.
This excellent evidence-based review summarized the various papers on nonsurgical treatment of de Quervain tenosynovitis. The only effective treatment was a targeted steroid injection.

Weiss AP, Akelman E, Tabatabai M. Treatment of de Quervain's disease. J Hand Surg Am 19:595, 1994.
This paper is more than 20 years old but is important, because it showed the greater efficacy of steroid injection versus splinting. The authors did not recommend splinting, because it was restrictive and without benefit.

82 Lateral Epicondylitis

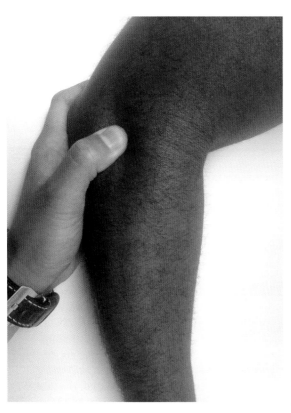

This 42-year-old executive developed right elbow pain after joining a tennis league 6 months ago.

Description of the Problem

The patient has pain centered over the area palpated on the lateral epicondyle (see photograph), with signs and symptoms of lateral epicondylitis.

Key Anatomy

Lateral epicondylitis, or tennis elbow, involves the forearm extensor muscles, specifically, the attachment of the extensor carpi radialis brevis (ECRB) on the lateral epicondyle. This causes pain with wrist extension and particularly with resisted wrist extension. It is an inflammation of this tendon-muscle origin and is exacerbated by repetitive activities such as playing tennis.

Workup

A history and a physical examination are critical for diagnosis. Often, patients have recently restarted playing tennis or have another new, strenuous activity such as painting a house or moving furniture. On an examination, the pain is centered on the lateral epicondyle. Patients note remarkable tenderness when this area is palpated. A careful palpation may reveal a step-off representing a partial tear of the ECRB insertion on the lateral epicondyle. Weakness of grip may be reported. Extension of the wrist against resistance will usually exacerbate the pain. Radiographs are obtained to rule out arthritis of the elbow. The initial treatment does not require an MRI; however, if lateral epicondylitis is resistant to conservative treatment, then an MRI may be helpful.

Treatment

The initial treatment is nonsurgical and usually successful. It includes rest by no longer participating in the same sports activities or heavy work activities for several weeks. Nonsteroidal antiinflammatory medications may help. Those who are focused on returning to tennis may need proper fitting of a racquet that will reduce stress on the forearm. Physical therapy modalities are important for improving healing of the ECRB origin. The most effective treatment is the use of a counterforce brace where the ECRB muscle is compressed more distally, thereby relieving pressure on the origin to allow healing of tendon to bone. Steroid injections may be useful if a brace is not successful.

Alternatives

Surgery is considered for patients in whom nonsurgical treatment is unsuccessful. It is rarely needed for this problem. It involves an open approach at the lateral epicondyle. The tendinosis of the ECRB is debrided, and the muscle is reattached to the bone with sutures. Arthroscopic debridement has been reported.

Principles and Clinical Pearls

- Pain on resisted wrist extension, point tenderness at the lateral epicondyle, and a history of a new, repetitive activity are highly suggestive of lateral epicondylitis.
- Conservative treatment comprising a change in activities, wearing a counterforce brace, stretching of the ECRB origin, and possible steroid injections is usually successful.
- Surgery is usually unnecessary, because most patients have resolution of symptoms with conservative measures.

Pitfalls

Pitfalls are related to inappropriate use of a counterforce brace. Many patients place the brace directly on the lateral epicondyle, which does not cause symptoms to resolve. It should be placed more distal to the lateral epicondyle. Steroid injections may cause further weakening of the insertion and/or discoloration of the skin. Aggressive surgical debridement may cause an open joint and continued egress of joint fluid in the region (and the development of a synoviocutaneous fistula). Haphazard excision has led to reports of injury to the posterior interosseous nerve and destabilization of the lateral aspect of the elbow by injury to the lateral ulnar collateral ligament.

Classic References

Szabo R. Steroid injection for lateral epicondylitis. J Hand Surg Am 34:326, 2009.
Doctor Szabo reviewed the evidence for and opinions about steroid injection for lateral epicondylitis. Based on the available data, the author concluded that no treatment has proved better than observation and behavior modification.

Wolf JM, Ozer K, Scott F, Gordon MJ, Williams AE. Comparison of autologous blood, corticosteroid, and saline injection in the treatment of lateral epicondylitis: a prospective, randomized, controlled multicenter study. J Hand Surg Am 36:1269, 2011.
In this prospective, blinded, randomized, controlled trial, the authors concluded that autologous blood and corticosteroid injection did not provide an advantage over saline injections. Conservative treatment with rest and behavior modification was usually the best treatment.

Tendon: Traumatic

83 Extensor Tendon Laceration

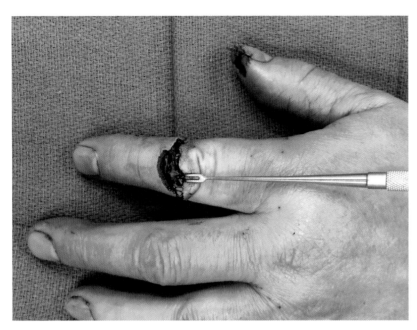

This patient is seen in the emergency department with a deep saw laceration to the dorsum of his left index finger.

Description of the Problem

The patient has extensive damage to the extensor tendon of the left index finger. His proximal interphalangeal joint is open. The finger is well vascularized.

Key Anatomy

The extensor tendon anatomy is much more complex than the flexor tendon anatomy. The central extensor tendon proceeds past the metacarpophalangeal joint to attach as the central slip onto the proximal portion of the middle phalanx. The lateral bands run on both sides of the central extensor tendon at the level of the proximal phalanx. They arise from the intrinsic muscles and continue past the central slip attachment to join together as the terminal extensor tendon, which extends the distal interphalangeal joint. The complex interplay between the lateral bands and the central slip is very difficult to re-create once it is injured. In this case, the laceration disrupted the central slip and opened the dorsal proximal interphalangeal joint.

Workup

Patients with an extensor tendon laceration should be assessed for active and passive range of motion to the proximal interphalangeal and distal interphalangeal joints. In this zone of injury, injury to the proximal interphalangeal joint itself should be suspected. The neurovascular status should also be carefully evaluated. Radiographs are obtained to look for joint involvement and bone involvement. Some have advocated repairing extensor tendons in the emergency room. However, we think that the complex nature of the extensor tendon anatomy warrants careful exploration and reconstruction in an operating room. This will lead to optimal results.

Treatment

The wound is well irrigated. Proximally and distally based skin flaps are elevated through midlateral incisions. Normal extensor tendon anatomy is found and traced into the level of the wound. The central extensor tendon and the lateral bands are identified. If the joint is involved, then intraoperative fluoroscopy may be useful to assess joint congruity. Most critical in an injury at this level is reconstruction of the central slip attachment to the middle phalanx. If the tendon is intact at the insertion, then a primary tendon repair can be performed. It is very important to separate the repair of the lateral bands from the central slip. If the central slip insertion has been obliterated, then a suture anchor may be used to reattach the central tendon to the base of the middle phalanx.

Alternatives

The alternative of repairing this injury in the emergency department exists; however, optimal results require careful exploration and repair in the operative room setting.

Principles and Clinical Pearls

- Extensor tendon anatomy is very complex and requires careful exploration and repair in an optimal setting.
- The central slip and the lateral bands control different joints, and their differences should be respected.
- Extensor tenolysis is frequently necessary after this repair. Early extensor tenolysis is essential, rather than stretching the thin extensor tendons with aggressive therapy. Once the extensor tendons are stretched, re-creating the normal pull of the tendons is very difficult.

Pitfalls

Pitfalls are related to detachment of the central slip and scarring of the lateral bands and central slip. Once these two separate structures are intermingled by scar, full extension and flexion of the digit are difficult to achieve. Cases of neglected central slip tendon injuries will present with chronic boutonnière deformities.

Classic References

Dy CJ, Rosenblatt L, Lee SK. Current methods and biomechanics of extensor tendon repairs. Hand Clin 29:261, 2013.
This was an excellent recent review of the biomechanics of extensor tendon repairs at each level. The authors specifically discussed central slip injuries.

Lutz K, Pipicelli J, Grewal R. Management of complications of extensor tendon injuries. Hand Clin 31:301, 2015.
Extensor tendons injuries are common, and their complications are widely seen. This article discussed the complications after these injuries.

Schubert CD, Giunta RE. Extensor tendon repair and reconstruction. Clin Plast Surg 41:525, 2014.
This review article focused on extensor tendon repair and reconstruction, including reconstruction of extensor tendon function with tendon lengthening, tendon grafts, tendon transfer, and coverage of large defects.

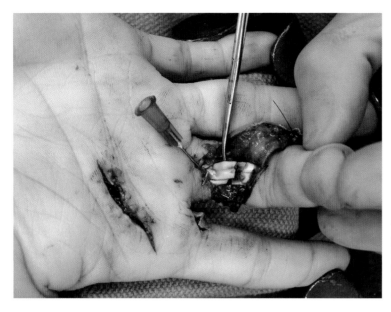

This 24-year-old office worker cut his left index finger on a knife while shucking oysters. He went to an emergency department, where his laceration was washed and closed. He is shown in the operating room 2 days later.

Description of the Problem

This patient has a severe laceration of the finger in zone II. Both the flexor digitorum profundus and the flexor digitorum superficialis are completely cut. In addition, the ulnar digital nerve and artery are cut.

Key Anatomy

Zone II is the region of the finger from the A1 pulley in the palm to just distal to the insertion of the flexor digitorum superficialis tendon. Both flexor tendons reside in the tight synovial sheath with a series of pulleys that prevent bow-stringing. This tight tunnel, which provides a biomechanical advantage for gliding, causes poor tendon gliding after flexor tendon repair. When both tendons are repaired, the bulk of the repair and the resulting scars lead to an inability to move the tendons.

Workup

Radiographs may be indicated if a fracture or foreign body is suspected. The workup consists of a detailed physical examination. The capillary refill and sensation are assessed. Then, the finger is tested for active flexion of the distal interphalangeal and proximal interphalangeal joints. Independent testing of these joints will help to determine whether one or both flexor tendons have been cut.

Treatment

Early exploration and repair of the cut structures are critical for easy, tension-free approximation. The digital nerve and artery are repaired under a microscope.

Much has been written about the optimal flexor tendon repair. Regardless of the technique chosen, several key principles should be followed. The incision is extended to allow retrieval of the flexor tendons. The A2 and A4 pulleys are identified, and at least part of them are preserved to prevent postoperative bow-stringing. As the flexor tendons are retrieved, the exact orientation of the two tendons is re-created. The flexor digitorum superficialis tendon starts on top, splits and turns sideways, and inserts onto the middle phalanx upside down. If this is not re-created, then excessive bulk will be present in relation to the flexor digitorum profundus tendon. The repair itself is performed with at least four-core sutures (preferably locking) and an epitendinous suture to make the edges neater. Both tendons should be repaired well and examined carefully to make sure gapping is not present. If the bulk of the repair is restricted by either the A2 or A4 pulley, a portion of the pulley can be "vented" or opened, while preserving some part of them.

The wound is closed meticulously, and a dorsal blocking splint is placed with the wrist neutral, the metacarpophalangeal joints flexed 90 degrees, and the interphalangeal joints extended. Splinting in excessive flexion is not necessary and only leads to flexion contractures. The patient is seen in the first few days after surgery to begin an early active motion protocol.

Alternatives

This zone II flexor tendon injury is a straightforward problem requiring immediate attention. If the flexor tendons are not repaired, then the tendon sheath and tendons will scar, requiring staged tendon reconstruction consisting of initial placement of a silicone rod and secondary tendon grafting. This alternative is not advisable.

Principles and Clinical Pearls

- The current optimal treatment is a flexor tendon repair with at least four-core suture strands.
- The A2 and A4 pulleys should be preserved, but a portion of them can be released to allow gliding of the repair.
- An early motion therapy protocol will promote better outcomes.

Pitfalls

This is a technically difficult procedure, because the margin for error is extremely narrow. A fine balance exists postoperatively between the two pitfalls of tendon rupture versus tendon adhesions. If the tendon ruptures, then an early exploration and rerepair are warranted; otherwise, staged tendon reconstruction is necessary. Poor active range of motion is probably related to tendon adhesions, and flexor tenolysis will be required.

Classic References

Chauhan AC, Palmer BA, Merrel GA. Flexor tendon repairs: techniques, eponyms, and evidence. J Hand Surg 39:1846, 2014.
The type of repair and the eponyms associated with each suture configuration are topics of great confusion. This was a nice review of the different suture techniques, accompanied by diagrams of each repair. The authors discussed the need for a four-strand or more repair technique to allow early active motion.

Trumble TE, Vedder NB, Seiler JG III, Hanel DP, Diao E, Pettrone S. Zone-II flexor tendon repair: a randomized prospective trial of active place-and-hold therapy compared with passive motion therapy. J Bone Joint Surg Am 92:1381, 2010.
This was an excellent multicenter prospective trial of zone II flexor tendon repairs. A passive motion therapy protocol was compared with an active motion therapy protocol. The active motion group had smaller flexion contractures and greater satisfaction scores. A certified hand therapist contributed to better results. This should be standard for postoperative management.

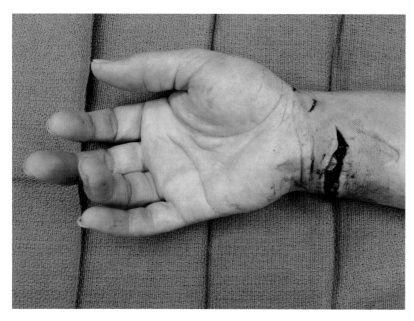

This 42-year-old woman has a deep laceration to her right volar wrist after falling onto a glass coffee table. She is seen in the emergency department.

Description of the Problem

This region of the wrist has many unprotected structures, including flexor tendons, the median and ulnar nerves, and the radial and ulnar arteries. Glass lacerations in this area can cause extensive damage. Exploration and repair are critical.

Key Anatomy

The volar distal wrist is relatively unprotected. The radial artery and ulnar artery are exposed. The median nerve and ulnar nerve are in the zone of injury. Other structures that can be injured include eight flexor tendons to the fingers, one flexor tendon to the thumb, and three flexor tendons to the wrist. The orientation of these tendons and nerves must be carefully evaluated so proper repair can be performed. If both the radial and the ulnar artery are cut, then the hand may be devascularized.

Workup

The patient is seen emergently, and a careful history is obtained to find the cause of the laceration. Usually, a sharp glass or knife injury has occurred. If a suicide attempt is suspected, then a psychiatric evaluation is obtained. The perfusion to the hand and sensation to the fingers are examined. The patient may have difficulty with flexion because of pain. Although this is not a surgical emergency, it is best to explore and repair the cut structures within 24 hours, because the nerves can begin to shorten. Nerve grafting may be necessary if treatment does not begin within a few days. If the hand shows signs of decreased blood flow, then the patient is taken emergently to the operating room. Usually, an angiogram is not necessary, because the vessels can be easily explored at this level.

Treatment

A precise technical order of repair makes this a 3-hour operation rather than a 6-hour operation. First, the hand is exsanguinated, and the tourniquet is inflated. The wound is copiously irrigated, with care to assess for glass shards in the wound. The transverse wrist incision is extended with midlateral incisions proximally and connected to a longitudinal carpal tunnel incision distally. A carpal tunnel incision is often necessary to expose the median nerve and the flexor tendons in the carpal canal.

The radial artery and the ulnar artery are the first structures examined and identified. If they are cut, they are temporarily clipped to facilitate identification. The median and ulnar nerves are similarly identified. The flexor tendon repair proceeds from deep to superficial and from radial to ulnar. Excess tenosynovium is removed, but the orientation of the flexor tendons is carefully preserved. If the flexor tendons are stripped too much, then re-creating the natural orientation of the flexor tendons will be difficult. Rather than identifying all the flexor tendons and then repairing them, we advocate repairing the flexor tendons "as you go" once they are identified.

Tendons are typically repaired with a four-strand Kessler repair. Epitendinous sutures are not needed. After the flexor pollicis longus tendon is treated, the flexor digitorum profundus tendons and flexor digitorum superficialis tendons are repaired, followed by the wrist flexors. The flexor carpi ulnaris tendon is the only flexor tendon that is not repaired before the nerves and arteries, because it lies superficial to the ulnar nerve and artery. With the tourniquet still inflated, the median and the ulnar nerve are carefully reapproximated by ensuring correct orientation of the fascicles. These nerves are repaired while the field remains bloodless.

After the flexor tendons and nerves are repaired, the tourniquet is let down and the proximal ends of the radial and ulnar arteries are identified. The proximal inflow is confirmed, and the microvascular anastomoses are performed. Surgeons should not forget to repair the flexor carpi ulnaris tendon, which can occur because they are preoccupied with the arterial repair. The skin is gently reapproximated. If the tension is too great, skin grafting on the midlateral areas is performed. A dorsal blocking splint is applied to prevent wrist and finger extension that may disrupt the repairs. In these cases, the hand is not completely devascularized; therefore time can be taken to precisely repair each tendon, nerve, and artery.

Alternatives

There are no alternatives to this emergent operation. It is critical to not delay this surgery, because identifying the cut structures later will be much more difficult.

Principles and Clinical Pearls

- Surgeons should anticipate that the laceration is deep and that multiple nerves, tendons, and arteries may have been cut.
- Repair in a precise order will allow facile and speedy reconstruction.
- We prefer to perform arterial anastomoses last, thereby operating in a bloodless field for most of the operation.

Pitfalls

The main pitfall is misidentification of tendons and nerves. It is easy to reconnect the wrong flexor tendons; therefore care is taken to properly identify and understand the topography of the flexor tendons. In addition, there may be scarring in this area, which will require future tenolysis and neurolysis.

Classic Reference

Noaman HH. Management and functional outcomes of combined injuries of flexor tendons, nerves, and vessels at the wrist. Microsurgery 27:536, 2007.
This was a retrospective review of 42 patients with spaghetti wrist lacerations over an 8-year period. The results were good to excellent for these complex injuries. One noted that median and ulnar nerve return was fairly good, because the injuries were distal.

86 Swan-Neck Deformity

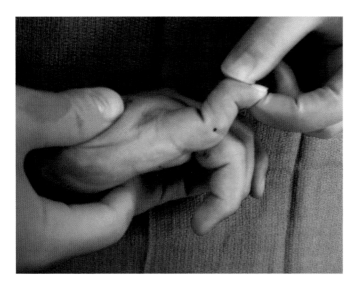

This 32-year-old woman has chronic hyperextension of the right small finger proximal interphalangeal (PIP) joint and flexion of the distal interphalangeal (DIP) joint. She is seen in the operating room before reconstruction.

Description of the Problem

The patient has a classic swan-neck deformity with DIP flexion and PIP joint hyperextension. It is critical to determine the cause of this deformity.

Key Anatomy

The extensor tendon complex and the contribution of the intrinsic muscles as lateral bands are a precisely organized series of forces. Any imbalance of the extrinsic and intrinsic forces can lead to characteristic deformities such as a swan-neck deformity. This deformity has three major causes. Congenital or traumatic volar plate laxity of the PIP joint leads to hyperextension of the PIP joint and resultant flexion of the DIP joint. Conversely, a chronic mallet finger with flexion of the DIP joint may compensate by hyperextension of the PIP joint. Third, in cases of intrinsic muscle tightness, the lateral bands will subluxate dorsal to the axis of the PIP joint rotation. The triangular ligament tightens, and the transverse retinacular ligament becomes lax, leading to increased force at the PIP joint with hyperextension of the joint and resultant flexion of the DIP joint.

Workup

A history is critical to determine whether the condition was caused by an inciting injury such as a mallet finger or a traumatic rupture of the volar plate to the PIP joint. The treatment is based on re-creating the anatomy that was present before the injury. A patient may have more systemic abnormalities such as rheumatoid arthritis. Patients are examined for passive and active range of motion. In some cases, the deformity may be fixed because of underlying bone or joint abnormalities. Furthermore, the capsule may be tight, leading to a fixed deformity. In patients with a dynamic deformity, the maximum flexion and extension arcs of each joint are measured. Maximal extension will accentuate the deformity. Radiographs are taken to assess for joint subluxation and arthritis.

Treatment

A trial of splinting may be employed; however, swan-neck deformities usually do not respond because of the degree of extensor tendon imbalance. Treatment is based on the underlying cause of the deformity. If it is caused by a chronic mallet finger, then the terminal extensor tendon can be advanced to correct the DIP joint and to provide more tendon length and tension at the PIP joint.

If the PIP joint volar plate is lax, two surgical options are available. Littler described the first procedure, which uses a slip of the flexor digitorum superficialis tendon. The proximal slip is detached and tethered to the proximal phalanx. This generates a volar force across the PIP joint that prevents hyperextension of the joint. Thompson described the second procedure for treating a lax volar plate. In this spiral oblique retinacular ligament reconstruction, a free tendon graft (commonly the palmaris longus tendon) is passed in a dorsal to volar direction through the base of the distal phalanx. The graft is routed through subcutaneous tissue deep to the neurovascular bundle along the side of the finger and then spiraled obliquely and volarly across the PIP joint to the opposite side of the finger. The tendon graft is routed through the base of the proximal phalanx. This sets the DIP joint in a neutral position and the PIP joint in slight flexion to create a flexion force at the PIP joint and an extension force at the DIP joint. This procedure is more complicated than the Littler superficialis tenodesis technique. Patients with a subluxated or abnormal joint may be better suited to PIP joint fusion.

Alternatives

Splinting and physical therapy are usually unsuccessful, because a swan-neck deformity is a chronic imbalance of the tendons. Treatment should start with the most conservative procedure—either reattachment of the terminal extensor tendon or a superficialis tenodesis—before more involved techniques are performed, such as the Thompson spiral oblique retinacular ligament reconstruction. Patients should be counseled that they may wish to avoid treatment, because it is very difficult to achieve satisfaction with a reconstruction.

Principles and Clinical Pearls

- A swan-neck deformity is described as hyperextension at the PIP joint and flexion at the DIP joint.
- Where the imbalance began and the cause need to be determined. Understanding the cause will help to choose an appropriate treatment. Swan-neck deformity may begin with pathology at either the MCP, PIP, or DIP joint.
- Surgery is based on re-creating the extensor tendon force at the DIP joint or creating a volar force at the PIP joint.

Pitfalls

Treatment has many pitfalls, because of the difficulty of re-creating the fine extensor tendon balance that previously existed. All of our techniques are crude, compared with the normal anatomy. Patients can have a recurrent abnormality, stiffness, and poor function after any of the procedures described previously.

Classic Reference

Smith GC, Amirfeyz R. The flexible swan neck deformity in rheumatoid arthritis. J Hand Surg Am 38:1405, 2013.
This was an excellent review of dynamic swan-neck deformities, especially in rheumatoid arthritis patients. The article described the various transfers that are possible for dynamic reconstruction.

87 Boutonnière Deformity

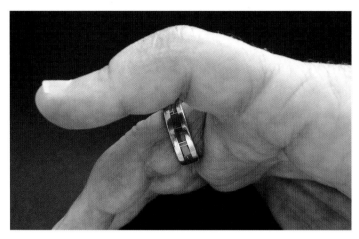

This 41-year-old man fell onto his left hand when it was in a fist position. He has swelling over the dorsum of the proximal interphalangeal (PIP) joint of his left small finger.

Description of the Problem

The patient has pain to the dorsum of his left small finger. He is unable to fully extend the finger at the PIP joint. He has some hyperextension of the distal interphalangeal (DIP) joint. This is consistent with an acute boutonnière deformity.

Key Anatomy

A boutonnière deformity involves DIP joint hyperextension and PIP joint flexion. The mechanism leading to this is usually disruption of the central slip from the base of the middle phalanx. The normal extensor tendon proceeds distally over the metacarpophalangeal joint and inserts as the central slip onto the base of the middle phalanx. This allows active extension of the PIP joint. Over time, if this injury is not treated, the transverse retinacular ligament contracts, and the lateral bands begin to displace volar to the PIP joint axis. They become shortened and fixed in this position. The patient is unable to passively extend the PIP joint, which leads to joint contractures, arthritic changes of the joint, and compensatory hyperextension at the DIP joint.

Workup

Patients with closed injuries of the PIP joint should be evaluated with radiographs. Those with no fracture or dislocation should be examined for full flexion and extension actively and passively. In some patients, disruption of the central slip is subtle and testing for active extension at the PIP joint with resistance is needed.

Treatment

The initial treatment of a closed boutonnière deformity consists of conservative management with extension splinting of the PIP joint and active motion at the DIP joint. When diagnosed early and splinted, a boutonnière deformity will usually respond to this management. The central slip will heal back to the middle phalanx, allowing resumption of a normal range of motion. A fixed deformity may result if the diagnosis is missed; this should first be treated with serial splinting and exercise before a surgical release. The goal is to alleviate flexion contracture of the PIP joint.

Late surgical correction of a boutonnière deformity is extremely difficult and should be reserved for patients who do not respond to splinting. Several procedures have been advocated, all of which attempt to divert the increased tone at the DIP joint in favor of the PIP joint. In a Fowler procedure, the extensor mechanism is approached through a dorsal incision distal to the PIP joint. The extensor mechanism is divided in a transverse direction at the junction of the middle and proximal third of the middle phalanx. The release allows the lateral bands to slide proximally, thus increasing tone over the PIP joint. At the same time, tone is relaxed over the DIP joint.

Alternatives

Alternatives to the Fowler procedure for chronic boutonnière deformity include the Littler procedure, in which the lateral bands are released and shifted dorsally and sutured to the central tendon, transforming the lateral bands into active extensors of the PIP joint. Alternatively, if a large central defect is present over the PIP joint, a tendon graft may be used to bridge the gap in the central slip.

Principles and Clinical Pearls

- A good understanding of the complex extensor tendon anatomy is critical to understanding a boutonnière deformity.
- The key deficit is disruption of the central slip. The central slip should be carefully preserved in all procedures related to the extensor tendon.
- Early recognition of a closed boutonnière injury and splinting will help to prevent the need for the complex and unpredictable chronic procedures discussed previously.

Pitfalls

Once the careful balance of the extensor mechanism is disrupted, re-creating normal function is extremely difficult. The procedures presented have very unpredictable outcomes. Pitfalls are related to an inability to fully flex and extend the PIP joint in a coordinated fashion. Fixed flexion or extension deformities may result.

Classic References

Merritt WH. Relative motion splint: active motion after extensor tendon injury and repair. J Hand Surg Am 39:1187, 2014.
Dr. Merritt has had a long-term interest in immediate controlled active motion splinting protocols. The rationale of relative motion was used to minimize long-term immobilization in favor of achieving full, active function quickly.

To P, Watson JT. Boutonniere deformity. J Hand Surg Am 36:139, 2011.
This review of boutonnière deformity described an evidence-based approach to this complex problem.

Zhang X, Yang L, Shao X, Wen S, Zhu H, Zhang Z. Treatment of bony boutonniere deformity with a loop wire. J Hand Surg Am 36:1080, 2011.
The authors described their technique for treating a dorsal avulsion fracture of the central slip. The adherence of bone to bone contact was critical for re-creating central slip biomechanics.

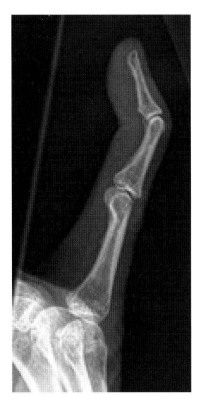

This patient jammed the tip of his small finger while playing softball.

Description of the Problem

No obvious fractures or dislocations are seen in this lateral radiograph. However, resting flexion is evident at the distal interphalangeal (DIP) joint. The patient is unable to extend his DIP joint actively. This is consistent with a soft tissue mallet finger.

Key Anatomy

The flexor tendons to the finger are thick and strong, whereas the extensor tendons are much thinner, and the terminal extensor tendon itself has a tenuous attachment to the distal phalanx. The terminal extensor tendon can easily be ruptured, resulting in a classic mallet finger whereby the flexor tendons overpower the absence of an extensor tendon insertion. The finger assumes a flexed posture. The proximal interphalangeal (PIP) joint may hyperextend in compensation.

Workup

Patients are usually seen in the clinic with a recent history of injury to the finger, swelling around the joint, some tenderness, and an inability to actively extend the finger. They may have already arrived with a temporary splint placed in the emergency department or by a primary care doctor. On an examination, active motion to the finger is assessed, and typically, patients cannot actively extend fully at the DIP joint. Radiographs are obtained to rule out a fracture at the distal phalanx, resulting in a bony mallet.

Treatment

Because the distal tendon is so wispy, surgery is not advised. Most patients do well with continuous hyperextension splinting at the DIP joint for 6 to 8 weeks. A special DIP joint extension splint is fashioned, which leaves the PIP joint free to perform active range of motion. Patients are checked at 4 weeks to ensure that they are following the instruction to leave the splint on at all times. The splint is then left in place for an additional 4 weeks. If a bony mallet is present, then splinting for a shorter length of time (4 to 6 weeks) is needed, because the bone will heal faster than the tendon insertion onto bone. After 8 weeks of continuous splinting, the splint is removed, and gentle, active range of motion therapy is begun.

Alternatives

Splinting may be useful even for mallet injuries that are several months old. However, for true chronic cases (longer than 1 year), some surgeons advocate an open advancement and repair of the tendon. Any surgery at this level is fraught with complications of stiffness, repair rupture, and infection. Some have advocated an indirect surgical approach. This involves division of the central slip attachment into the base of the middle phalanx, thus retensioning the lateral bands to exert their extension force at the level of the distal phalanx.

Principles and Clinical Pearls

- A mallet finger injury is based on an imbalance between the flexor tendon insertion and the extensor tendon insertion. The extensor tendon insertion is much more fragile and prone to rupture.
- Radiographs are necessary to rule out a fracture fragment or subluxation of the joint.
- Conservative treatment is best. This involves a 6- to 8-week period of DIP joint extension splinting, leaving the PIP joint free.

Pitfalls

Pitfalls include a poorly fashioned splint, which allows some flexion within the splint. If the PIP joint is also splinted, then stiffness of that joint may become evident after immobilization. The splint should be fashioned in a precise way to mimic hyperextension of the DIP joint. Surgery can result in the complications noted previously.

Classic References

Bloom J, Khouri J, Hammert W. Current concepts in the evaluation and treatment of mallet finger injury. Plast Reconstr Surg 133:891, 2014.
This was an excellent recent review of mallet finger injury, including splinting versus surgery.

Wada T, Oda T. Mallet fingers with bone avulsion and DIP joint subluxation. J Hand Surg Eur Vol 40:8, 2015.
The authors specifically addressed mallet fractures with a large fracture fragment that result in volar subluxation of the distal phalanx. These may require surgery versus nonoperative treatment. The authors proposed an extension block pinning technique for optimal surgery if necessary.

89 Flexor Tendon Avulsion

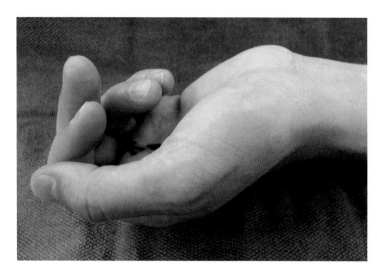

This 22-year-old college rugby player injured his left middle finger while grabbing a jersey.

Description of the Problem

The patient has an avulsion of the flexor digitorum profundus (FDP) tendon. These injuries require timely treatment to reinsert the flexor tendon at the distal phalanx level. His inability to flex his distal interphalangeal (DIP) joint is evident in the photograph.

Key Anatomy

The flexor digitorum superficialis (FDS) tendon splits and inserts onto the base of the middle phalanx. The FDP tendon progresses distally through this split and inserts onto the distal phalanx. Therefore the FDP tendon allows DIP joint flexion. In avulsion injuries, the FDP tendon is torn off of the distal phalanx. Leddy and Packer have proposed a straightforward classification that determines treatment based on the level of tendon retraction and the presence of a distal phalanx fracture. In type 1, the FDP tendon is retracted all the way into the palm. The vascular supply is disrupted. Prompt treatment with surgery is necessary within a week to prevent shortening of the muscle-tendon unit. In type 2, the FDP tendon retracts to the level of the proximal interphalangeal (PIP) joint. Repair as early as possible is prudent to prevent shortening. Type 3 is characterized by a large avulsion fracture from the distal phalanx that limits the retraction to the level of the DIP joint. Early repair is best; however, this can be more easily reattached to the bone, because the tendon is not shortened. Type 4 has a separate fracture fragment and simultaneous avulsion of the tendon from the fragment. This requires fixation of the fracture and reattachment of the tendon. Type 4 injuries are rare. The most commonly involved finger is the ring finger, because it is more prominent with gripping.

Workup

Patients with a finger injury and a suspected FDP avulsion should undergo active and passive range of motion testing. The passive flexion of the DIP joint should be full, but active flexion is limited. Tenderness and swelling along the sheath is possible, and type 1 injuries may have a tender nodule in the palm at the site of the tendon retraction. PIP joint active and passive motion should be full. A lateral radiograph may help to show the fracture fragment. Patient consent should be obtained for a wide range of treatment options from reinsertion to staged tendon reconstruction.

Treatment

Avulsion injuries should be treated as soon as possible so the tendon sheath remains patent with good room for gliding. The finger is approached through a Bruner incision from distal to proximal. Blood in the sheath will help to determine the level of injury. The tendon sheath is exposed distal to the A4 pulley, and the site of avulsion is identified. Dissection distally along the distal phalanx is critical so that it can be reattached as distal as possible. Depending on the level of the flexor tendon avulsion, counterincisions may need to be made to retrieve the flexor tendon. Great care is taken to prevent injury to the FDS tendon. Several options are available for reattachment of an avulsed FDP tendon. The simplest is a pullout wire with a button on the dorsum of the nail. Some authors have advocated miniscrew fixation or a suture anchor. One risk of using a suture anchor is that the fixation may be too proximal to provide a good moment arm for active flexion of the finger.

Alternatives

In chronic cases in which a flexor tendon sheath is no longer available, a staged flexor tendon reconstruction with re-creation of a tendon sheath using a Hunter rod can be performed. Alternatively, DIP joint arthrodesis may stabilize the DIP joint, obviating the need for a staged tendon reconstruction.

Principles and Clinical Pearls

- The Leddy-Packer classification for FDP avulsion injuries is very helpful in determining the level of injury and optimal timing of treatment.
- Reattachment of the FDP tendon as distal as possible onto the distal phalanx is essential to ensure a good moment arm for active flexion.
- Although DIP active flexion is useful, preserving PIP joint flexion is more critical, because salvage procedures such as DIP arthrodesis are effective for controlling the digit.

Pitfalls

Excessive advancement and shortening of the flexor tendon (more than 1 cm) can lead to the development of quadriga, in which the flexor tendons to the other fingers are tethered by the shortening. Any operation within the flexor tendon sheath risks increased scar and adhesion formation.

Classic References

Freilich AM. Evaluation and treatment of jersey finger and pulley injuries in athletes. Clin Sports Med 34:151, 2015.
This was an excellent recent review of the evaluation and treatment of jersey finger injuries, especially in athletes.

Lee S, Fajardo M, Kardashian G, Klein J, Tsai P, Christoforou D. Repair of flexor digitorum profundus to distal phalanx: a biomechanical evaluation of four techniques. J Hand Surg Am 36:1604, 2011.
Dr. Lee and his colleagues evaluated four different repair techniques for the FDP tendon to the distal phalanx. They suggested that the anchor technique may be a useful new development.

Yeh P, Shin SS. Tendon ruptures: mallet, flexor digitorum profundus. Hand Clin 28:425, 2012.
This was a review of tendon ruptures on both sides, the flexor tendon side and the extensor tendon side.

90 Flexor Tendon Adhesions

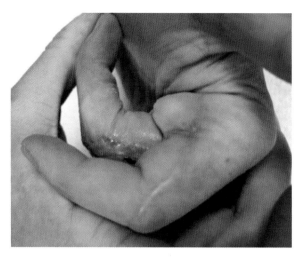

This 42-year-old man presents to the office after a repair of zone 2 flexor tendon lacerations of his middle finger flexor digitorum superficialis (FDS) and flexor digitorum profundus (FDP) tendons. After the repair, the patient followed a synergistic wrist motion protocol, and the splint was discontinued after 6 weeks. He had 3 more months of supervised therapy and was able to flex the finger actively to only 45 degrees of a total arc. With passive motion, the finger flexed to 80 degrees. He sought a consultation for evaluation of the state of his repair.

Description of the Problem

Fingers that have undergone repair of intrasynovial flexor tendon lacerations or repair of FDP avulsions from the base of the distal phalanx and have not achieved full, active digital flexion during the period of supervised therapy after the injury are at risk of one of three complications: a tendon rupture, a repair site elongation, and the formation of intrasynovial adhesions. Although tendons in continuity and those that have ruptured or elongated may possibly be differentiated in a clinical examination, this distinction can be confirmed only during a surgical exploration.

Key Anatomy

The fibrous flexor sheath begins at the A1 pulley at the level of the metacarpal head and the volar plate of the metacarpophalangeal joint and terminates at the A5 pulley at the level of the distal interphalangeal joint. Both the FDS and the FDP tendons enter the sheath at the origin. Deep to the A2 pulley, the FDS tendon bifurcates, rotates around the FDP tendon, joins back together over the proximal aspect of the volar shaft of the middle phalanx, and inserts on the central three fifths of the shaft of the middle phalanx, deep to the A4 pulley, as two slips. An important characteristic of the fibrous flexor sheath is that it is not distensible to any great extent, and swelling therein can limit motion, cause tendon repair site dehiscence, and increase the likelihood of the development of restrictive adhesions.

Workup

Imaging is not useful. Passive flexion, active flexion, passive extension, and active extension of the finger are precisely documented. If passive finger flexion is full but active flexion is incomplete, then the limitation to motion is sought within the fibrous flexor sheath. Dorsal adhesions or stiffness is not necessarily a concern if passive flexion is full.

Treatment

The fibrous flexor sheath is surgically explored through the zone of injury and proximal and distal to it. A tendon rupture or a repair site elongation may be encountered. In this case, the surgeon should be prepared for a re-repair (which is needed infrequently) or either a primary tendon graft (which is needed infrequently and only if the pulley system is intact and unblemished) or implantation of a silicone rod to create a new gliding surface, followed by tendon grafting on a delayed basis. If the tendon is found to be intact on exploration and only limited in excursion by the formation of intrasynovial adhesions, then a tenolysis is performed, followed by active motion therapy to maintain the gliding surface and the relative motion between the tendon and the sheath.

Alternatives

Nonoperative treatment might be favored for patients who can tolerate the degree of motion loss (especially on the radial side of the hand).

Principles and Clinical Pearls

- A flexor tendon repair can rupture up to 12 weeks postoperatively. Although flexor tendon repair site elongation occurs in the presence of distal adhesions, it can occur in the complete absence of adhesions and can result in acute motion loss during a seemingly successful therapeutic protocol.
- Patients should be informed preoperatively that the findings during exploration of the fibrous flexor sheath might require as many as three additional operations: a pulley reconstruction and silicone rod implantation, a delayed tendon graft, and a flexor tenolysis of the graft. For patients who are not prepared to undergo these procedures, suitable plans should be made for a backup procedure such as distal interphalangeal joint fusion and FDS-only grafting.

Pitfalls

Therapy after a re-repair or grafting requires finesse: Too much proximal musculotendinous load leads to rupture of the repair, and too little intrasynovial repair site excursion invites the formation of adhesion. As Johnny Cash said, "I walk the line."

Classic Reference

Jupiter JB, Goldfarb CA, Nagy L, Boyer MI. Posttraumatic reconstruction in the hand. J Bone Joint Surg Am 89:428, 2007.
The authors summarized the different algorithms useful for the surgical treatment of stiff fingers.

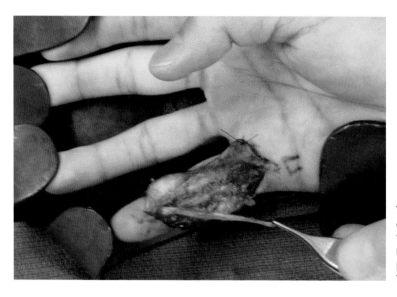

This patient is seen intraoperatively after exploration and tenolysis of a right small finger flexor tendon repair. No pulleys remain, and the small flexor digitorum profundus (FDP) tendon (held within the forceps) is scarred and transected.

Description of the Problem

The patient's small finger has no FDP or flexor digitorum superficialis (FDS) tendons and no pulleys. A staged flexor tendon reconstruction is required to re-create active flexion of the small finger.

Key Anatomy

The FDS and FDP tendons control active flexion of the proximal interphalangeal (PIP) and distal interphalangeal (DIP) joints. Once tendons scar, the normal gliding necessary for active flexion is difficult. The annular pulleys, specifically the A2 and A4 pulleys, are critical to prevent bow-stringing. In this case, staged tendon reconstruction is necessary.

Workup

This is a very difficult staged reconstruction procedure fraught with complications and shortcomings. First, the patient must be motivated to undergo a year-long protocol required to restore active flexion. The patient will be followed in physical therapy, with documentation of compliance. Those who do not reliably go to therapy before the operation probably will not do so afterward. In addition, all evidence of infection and exposed wounds must be addressed before the first stage.

An evaluation of the patient's passive range of motion is also essential. If the finger is stiff in extension, then an extensor tenolysis and capsulotomy should first be performed. The finger should be passively flexible before reconstruction. Radiographs are obtained to rule out joint subluxation or arthritis, which will limit the overall result. The patient should be counseled carefully regarding the likelihood that the reconstruction may not be satisfactory.

Treatment

In the first stage of treatment, the wound is opened along Bruner or midaxial incisions, and all scarred, useless flexor tendon is removed. A tendon graft is harvested that will be used for reconstructing the A2 and A4 pulleys. The grafts are woven around the middle phalanx and proximal phalanx and sewn to the base. This is done over a Hunter rod sizer.

A properly sized Hunter rod is placed and sutured distally to remaining FDP tendon or anchored to the distal phalanx bone. Proximally, the Hunter rod goes across the palm and into the distal forearm. It is left free to allow gliding. The wound is carefully closed to prevent infection, and passive range of motion is initiated.

The second stage begins 3 to 6 months after the first stage. The following prerequisites are confirmed before proceeding with the second stage:
- A lateral radiograph shows the Hunter rod remains in place.
- The finger has full, passive flexion.
- A soft, compliant soft tissue bed is present, with no open wounds.
- The patient is motivated.

The very distal part of the incision over the DIP joint is opened, and the very proximal part of the incision in the distal wrist is opened. The Hunter rod is identified and isolated at both ends. Most of the finger is not opened.

A tendon graft is harvested, either the palmaris longus tendon or a toe extensor. This tendon graft is then passed from proximal to distal by suturing it to the Hunter rod and then withdrawing the rod distally. The tendon graft is affixed to the distal phalanx either by sewing it to the remaining stump of FDP tendon or by placing it into the bone of the distal phalanx using a pullout wire. We prefer to test this distal coaptation by pulling proximally on the tendon graft at the wrist level.

The proximal end of the tendon graft is sutured in a Pulvertaft weave to either the FDP tendon of the ring finger or to a transferred FDS tendon from the ring finger. Suturing to a separate FDS tendon allows independent motion and prevents the risk of a lumbrical plus deformity or quadriga. The patient is given wide-awake anesthesia with lidocaine and epinephrine for the second stage. This allows active flexion of the small finger to test the tension to the transfer. Specific, graded active range of motion exercises are initiated in therapy.

Alternatives

In this case, both the FDP and FDS tendons are not present; therefore the patient has no active flexion across the PIP and DIP joints. In cases in which the FDS tendon is intact but the FDP tendon is missing, we would not advocate performing a staged tendon reconstruction for re-creation of DIP joint flexion only. This is an extraordinarily difficult and unreliable procedure, and the PIP active motion may possibly be limited afterward. These patients do well with either no treatment to the DIP joint or with a tenodesis/arthrodesis to control the joint.

Principles and Clinical Pearls

- Staged flexor tendon reconstruction is one of the most challenging procedures to obtain a good result. The patient and surgeon must be motivated to embark on a 1-year odyssey together.
- Obtaining a lateral radiograph of the finger after the first stage is critical to ensure that the Hunter rod has not migrated.
- Wide-awake anesthesia using lidocaine and epinephrine is an excellent technique for stage 2, because it allows the patient to participate in tensioning of the staged tendon graft reconstruction.

Pitfalls

There are many pitfalls to this prodedure. These include infection of the Hunter rod, tendon graft rupture, quadriga (if the tendon reconstruction is too tight), a lumbrical plus deformity (if there is remaining scarred FDP tendon that pulls the finger into extension), and recurrent scarring.

Classic Reference

Boyes JH, Stark HH. Flexor-tendon grafts in the fingers and thumb. A study of factors influencing results in 1000 cases. J Bone Joint Surg Am 53:1332, 1971.

This was the classic article describing staged tendon reconstruction.

Tumors

92 Mucous Cyst

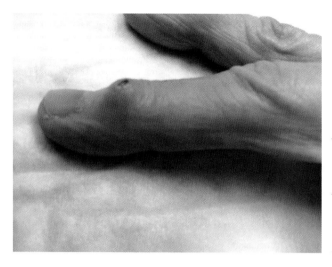

This 68-year-old woman presents with a painless, enlarging mass over the dorsoradial aspect of her middle finger distal interphalangeal (DIP) joint. It has been present for 4 months. The patient punctured the mass once to express clear gelatinous fluid, and it recurred within days. She notes a flattening of her nail plate immediately distal to the mass. DIP motion is active between 10 and 55 degrees. The sensation and neurovascular supply to the fingertip are normal.

Description of the Problem

A mucous cyst is a ganglion cyst of the DIP joint and is associated with underlying degenerative arthritis. A differential diagnosis includes a giant cell tumor and an epidermal inclusion cyst.

Key Anatomy

The cyst emanates from the dorsal aspect of the DIP joint and often compresses the germinal matrix of the nail. The overlying skin is frequently thinned.

Workup

PA and lateral plain radiographs and ultrasound (if a solid lesion is suspected or if the diagnosis is in question) are obtained.

Treatment

Mucous cysts can be treated nonoperatively with massage of the fluid back into the joint unless surgical removal is directly indicated. These indications include septic arthritis, a recurrent paronychia, pain, recurrent drainage, a progressive nail deformity, and aesthetic displeasure. Several techniques are available; however, all involve excision of the underlying bony osteophyte, which usually emanates from the base of the distal phalanx. The joint cyst is completely excised with or without the overlying skin. The cyst wall need not be sent for pathologic examination. If a large defect is present, a local skin flap can be rotated to cover the defect, and a full-thickness skin graft can be placed on the flap harvest site. Dressings are kept in place for 2 weeks, and early active and active-assisted range of motion are initiated once the wound is stable.

Alternatives

Some surgeons recommend osteophyte removal only. The cyst involutes as a result.

Principles and Clinical Pearls

- Total excision of a cyst and cyst wall requires exposure of the nail plate, the sterile matrix, and the dorsal aspect of the eponychial fold. Injury of these structures can cause permanent nail deformity.
- The cyst is in direct communication with the DIP joint. A draining cyst is therefore an open joint and has the potential for becoming a septic joint.
- Joint fusion is required infrequently.

Pitfalls

Surgical excision may result in recurrence, wound dehiscence, infection of the joint or soft tissue, flap necrosis, skin graft necrosis, stiffness, or pain. Patient expectations should be tempered preoperatively.

Classic Reference

Fritz GR, Stern PJ, Dickey M. Complications following mucous cyst excision. J Hand Surg Br 22:222, 1997.
After excision of 86 mucous cysts in 79 patients, the following complications were noted: extension loss of up to 20 degrees, superficial infection, DIP septic arthritis, nail deformities that did not resolve, new nail deformities not present preoperatively, recurrence, swelling, pain, frontal plane deformity, paresthesias, and stiffness. The authors recommended a preoperative discussion of these possible risks of this seemingly straightforward procedure.

93 Dorsal Wrist Ganglion

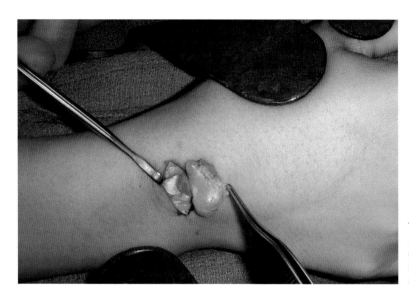

This 23-year-old woman is undergoing excision of a right wrist dorsal ganglion. She initially presented with dorsal pain and swelling. The mass was aspirated twice, but it recurred.

Description of the Problem

The patient presented with a dorsal wrist mass. The differential diagnosis includes a dorsal wrist ganglion, extensor tenosynovitis, less common benign tumors such as inclusion cysts and lipomas, and rare, anomalous anatomic variants such as the extensor digitorum brevis manus muscle. A circumscribed mass that fluctuates in size over time is most likely a dorsal wrist ganglion. This diagnosis is confirmed if a characteristic viscous, clear fluid is aspirated.

Key Anatomy

Understanding the anatomy of a dorsal wrist ganglion is critical for successful treatment. These lesions nearly always emanate from the scapholunate ligament dorsally and cause a herniation of the dorsal wrist capsule. Synovial fluid from the wrist leaks into the ganglion cavity and cannot return because of a valvelike mechanism. Therefore a dorsal wrist ganglion can increase or decrease in size. Aspiration may not be successful in the long term, because the cyst's lining is not removed. Surgical excision involves removing the entire cyst lining and tracking the stalk of the ganglion into the wrist joint. A portion of the wrist capsule is removed with great care not to damage the scapholunate ligament. Smaller, occult cysts can actually cause more pain than larger ones by pressing on the overlying posterior interosseous nerve. Cyst removal and/or removal of the distal end of the posterior interosseous nerve usually relieves pain.

Workup

The workup for a dorsal wrist ganglion is very simple. A fluctuating increase and decrease in the size of the cyst is confirmed. A clear, viscous aspirate is pathognomonic for a dorsal wrist ganglion. Radiographs are usually unnecessary unless the lesion causes significant wrist pain, which could signify an underlying scapholunate ligament issue. In patients who have dorsal wrist pain at the site of the scapholunate ligament with no mass and negative radiographs, an MRI or ultrasound may be indicated to assess for an occult ganglion pressing on the posterior interosseous nerve.

Treatment

Treatment for a dorsal wrist ganglion usually begins with aspiration, which can be performed as many times as necessary. However, complete removal is unlikely, because the cyst lining remains. Open surgery is indicated if the ganglion recurs and is bothersome to the patient. The mass does not need to be removed if the patient does not wish it. The surgery is straightforward. A transverse incision is made over the dorsal wrist at the level of the scapholunate ligament. This incision is used because it heals with less scarring. The extensor tendons are identified and protected. Dissection proceeds circumferentially around the cyst. Careful dissection of the ganglion without puncturing it will facilitate identification of the underlying stalk. Removing a portion of the wrist capsule provides an opening into the wrist joint. The scapholunate ligament is again protected. Once the cyst is removed, bleeding branches of the posterior interosseous artery are controlled with bipolar cautery. The incision is closed with subcuticular sutures to minimize scarring.

Alternatives

The historical alternative was to hit the mass with a Bible or another heavy book to pop it. Some surgeons now advocate arthroscopic ganglion removal as an alternative to an open excision.

Principles and Clinical Pearls

- Less likely diagnoses for a dorsal wrist mass should be considered, including extensor tenosynovitis and benign tumors.
- Surgery is straightforward and recurrence rates are low if the ganglion is removed circumferentially and the stalk is tracked to the level of the dorsal wrist capsule.
- An occult ganglion is suspected in patients with dorsal wrist pain with no evidence of a mass.

Pitfalls

Pitfalls include poor resection of the stalk and wrist capsule leading to recurrence and damage to the underlying scapholunate ligament. The wrist should be immobilized for only a short time to prevent stiffness.

Classic References

Ahsan ZS, Yao J. Arthroscopic dorsal wrist ganglion excision with color-aided visualization of the stalk: minimum 1-year follow-up. Hand 9:205, 2014.
The authors described the technique of arthroscopic ganglionectomy using dye injection.

McKeon K, Boyer MI, Goldfarb CA. Use of routine histologic evaluation of carpal ganglions. J Hand Surg Am 31:284, 2006.
In a large series of volar and dorsal wrist ganglion excisions, the authors showed that results of pathology evaluations were extremely likely to be as predicted—benign. Therefore they rightly questioned the need for and cost of sending specimens for histologic review.

94 Glomus Tumor

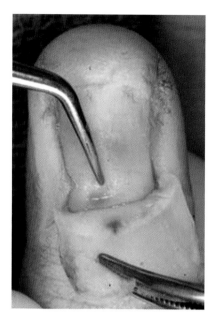

This patient is shown intraoperatively with a circumscribed lesion just underneath the nail bed. The patient had exquisite pain in the region for several years before the workup and treatment.

Description of the Problem

A glomus tumor is a tumor of the neuromyovascular system that arises typically underneath the nail bed in the finger. Patients can have excruciating pain in this area and pain with temperature changes. Often, the tumor is misdiagnosed, because patients have the unusual symptom of extreme pain in a fingertip with negative plain radiographs.

Key Anatomy

The cell type that causes this tumor is the glomus cell. These are specialized smooth muscle cells derived from pericytes that control vasodilation. They arise from the neuromyoarterial system and are thought to control temperature regulation in the finger. As a mass begins to grow underneath the nail, it causes extreme pain out of proportion to its size. The typical location is underneath the nail just distal to the germinal matrix.

Workup

Patients are seen in the hand clinic with exquisite tenderness to the tip of the finger. Radiographs are usually performed and do not reveal abnormalities. Osteoarthritis and bone spurs at the level of the distal interphalangeal joint are ruled out. If extreme pain at the site of the fingernail continues, then the fingernail is inspected for color changes and other abnormalities. The index of suspicion for a glomus tumor should be high in patients with extreme pain at the fingertip. An MRI usually reveals a small circumscribed lesion.

Treatment

Glomus tumors are treated with surgical excision. In most cases, the nail itself must be gently removed, and a longitudinal incision is made in the nail bed and the tumor is removed. Hemostasis is confirmed, and the nail bed is carefully reapproximated with absorbable suture. The nail is replaced to splint the proximal nail fold open so that the new nail can grow over this lesion. The nail bed should not be removed; otherwise, complex nail bed reconstruction is required.

Alternatives

Several alternatives to surgical treatment are available. Most pertain to the differential diagnoses, including osteoarthritis of the distal interphalangeal joint and neuroma formation.

Principles and Clinical Pearls

- Glomus tumors are rare, commonly misdiagnosed masses that cause extraordinary pain.
- The surgery is very delicate to allow removal of the mass without significantly damaging the underlying nail bed.
- An MRI is the optimal imaging study to localize the mass.

Pitfalls

The greatest pitfall is a misdiagnosis, leading to continued pain. Haphazard surgery can damage the nail bed to the extent that the proximal nail will not grow, and the nail will never be completely normal again. The mass can recur.

Classic References

Gandhi J, Yang SS, Hurd J. The anatomic location of digital glomus tumor recurrences. J Hand Surg Am 35:986, 2010.
This group reviewed the anatomic locations of recurrent glomus tumors. All recurrent tumors occurred in new, separate locations from the original lesions, suggesting that inadequate resection is not the cause of recurrence.

McDermott EM, Weiss AP. Glomus tumors. J Hand Surg Am 31:1397, 2006.
This was an excellent review showing surgical techniques for excision.

Yanai T, Tanaka T, Ogawa T. Immunohistochemical demonstration of cyclooxygenase-2 in glomus tumors. J Bone Joint Surg Am 95:725, 2013.
Eight primary glomus tumors were stained and found to be positive for S100 protein and cyclooxygenase-2. Substance P was found in five of the eight samples. The cyclooxygenase-2–prostaglandin E2 pathway may control the vasodilation seen at the fingertip.

95 Hemangioma

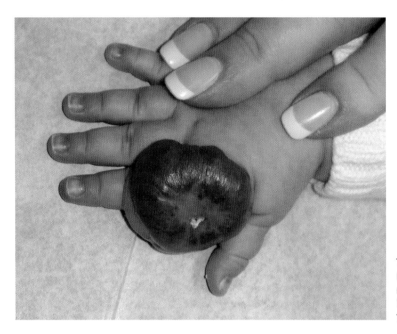

This 18-month-old child is seen in the hand clinic with a mass involving her right hand. It was a small mass at birth but has expanded in size in the past year.

Description of the Problem

The child has a mass on the right hand that may be a hemangioma or a vascular malformation. Diagnosing the lesion based on a history and physical examination is critical, because the treatment for a hemangioma versus a vascular malformation is very different. A hemangioma will increase in size in the first years of life but will involute or shrink by around 7 years of age. A vascular malformation is present at birth and grows proportionately with the child.

Key Anatomy

The mass involves the dorsum of the index finger, the first web space, and the volar aspect of the index finger, extending into the palm. It is a soft tissue tumor, but it may involve the deeper structures and even deform the bone. Planning for a surgical excision requires consideration of the need for complex reconstruction with grafts and flaps.

Workup

Such lesions are best diagnosed with a careful history regarding the timing of growth, which facilitates identification as either a hemangioma or a vascular malformation. The extent of the growth and vascular involvement can be assessed with an MR angiogram.

Treatment

Hemangiomas generally involute over time. Indications for early excision of hemangiomas are limited to bleeding, ulceration, and/or infection. The residual mass, which is usually some excess fatty skin, can be excised electively. If the mass is a vascular malformation, then the first step is to determine whether it is amenable to resection. The mass is palpated for a thrill and auscultated for a bruit, which would be present in high-flow arterial malformations. These can be life-threatening and very difficult to control. Slow-flow venous malformations may distort normal anatomy and infiltrate vessels throughout an area. Vascular malformations commonly recur if not excised completely. However, complete resection may damage critical structures.

Alternatives

Hemangiomas are occasionally treated with local steroid injections. A systemic steroid or propranolol treatment is reserved for more threatening hemangiomas on the face and periorbital area. Nonsurgical treatment of vascular malformations begins with compression garments. If the lesion is extensive and surgery would be difficult, both sclerotherapy and embolization can be performed. As in all surgeries, these procedures have significant risks, including recurrence, wound breakdown, and ischemia.

Principles and Clinical Pearls

- The most critical, first step is diagnosing the lesion as either a hemangioma or a vascular malformation. These two masses are very different, with different outcomes and treatment plans.
- Hemangiomas usually involute and do not need surgical treatment unless ulceration, infection, or bleeding is a concern.
- Surgery is undertaken for vascular malformations only if the chance for complete excision is reasonable. Surgeons should anticipate a complex resection requiring microsurgical dissection.
- In many cases, surgery is not attempted, because adequate resection would lead to loss of digital function.

Pitfalls

Incomplete resection will probably lead to recurrence. On the other hand, complete resection has the significant risks of bleeding, skin loss, and ischemia, resulting in amputation.

Classic References

Marqueling AL, Oza V, Frieden IJ, Puttgen KB. Propranolol and infantile hemangiomas four years later: a systematic review. Pediatr Dermatol 30:182, 2013.
There is tremendous interest in the use of propranolol for nonsurgical treatment of hemangiomas. This systematic review spanned from 2008 to 2012. The response rate for patients with hemangiomas treated with propranolol was a remarkable 98%, with response rate loosely defined as any improvement with propranolol. With this efficacy, propranolol has become the first-line treatment for hemangiomas in need of early treatment.

Willard KJ, Cappel MA, Kozin SH, Abzug JM. Congenital and infantile skin lesions affecting the hand and upper extremity, part 1: vascular neoplasms and malformations. J Hand Surg Am 38:2271, 2013.
This was an excellent recent review of vascular anomalies of the hand. The differences between hemangiomas and vascular malformations were outlined, and treatment algorithms were presented.

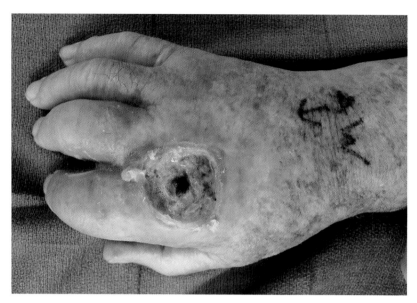

This 76-year-old man presents to his primary care doctor with a 9-month history of a steadily enlarging mass over the dorsum of his right hand. He has no history of trauma. He worked as a truck driver in the Southwest for 35 years before retiring 9 years ago. The mass is painless, nonpruritic, and fixed to the underlying tissue. It has a scaly surface and bleeds with minor trauma. The patient has no systemic symptoms and no lymphadenopathy at his elbow or in his axilla.

Description of the Problem

Squamous cell carcinoma of the skin can occur anywhere on the body but has a predilection for sun-damaged areas of skin. It is a slow-growing tumor with little propensity to metastasize; however, local control by surgical excision with clear margins (both deep and at the periphery of the lesion) is necessary.

Key Anatomy

Local drainage of the hand through lymphatics would carry cells to the supratrochlear lymph node at or above the elbow and to the axillary lymph nodes deep to the pectoralis major or the latissimus dorsi muscles, along the chest wall or along the medial aspect of the proximal humerus.

Workup

Biopsy and excision are typically the only workup needed. Additional studies to assess for metastatic disease are required infrequently. If necessary, standard imaging studies include chest and abdominal CT scans and plain radiographs of the affected area to assess for bone destruction. Primary squamous cell cancer of the lung has a propensity to acrometastasis, that is, to spread to the distal phalanges. It can mimic a felon or osteomyelitis of the distal phalanx (see Chapter 59), and a biopsy should be performed at the time of surgical treatment of the fingertip mass.

Treatment

Treatment consists of excision and confirmation of tumor-free margins. Local flap coverage and a skin graft may be needed. Larger defects can require local perforator or axial-pattern flaps to be rotated to cover exposed structures. Useful flaps that can be rotated locally include an ulnar artery perforator flap, a posterior interosseous artery flap, and a reverse pedicle radial forearm flap (either with or without concurrent harvest of the radial artery.)

Alternatives

Local treatment with chemotherapeutic agents is an option for patients who are unable or unwilling to have surgical excision. Squamous cell cancer occurring within the sterile or germinal nail matrix can be treated by amputation or disarticulation.

Principles and Clinical Pearls

- Mohs surgery is the most frequently used treatment modality for superficial squamous cell cancers of the dorsum of the hand.
- Dorsal rotation flaps can be performed easily in elderly patients who have redundancy of dorsal tissue that is suitable for the construction of adjacent flaps.
- For patients with a risk of metastasis, a medical oncologist can perform staging before or after excision of the mass.

Pitfalls

Pitfalls include inadequate excision or insufficient tissue for local closure options.

Classic Reference

Askari M, Kakar S, Moran SL. Squamous cell carcinoma of the hand: a 20-year review. J Hand Surg Am 38:2124, 2013.
This retrospective review outlined the risk of metastasis (4%) and local recurrence based on the characteristics of the local tumor. Factors that favored local recurrence included location of the tumor in a web space, bilateral tumors, positive history of a prior squamous cell carcinoma, and the presence of multiple tumors. The authors found no significant effect of Mohs resection on either local recurrence or survival.

97 Melanoma

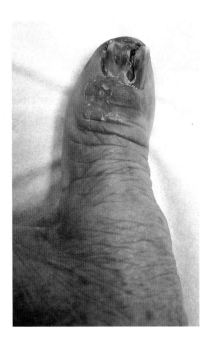

This patient is seen in the clinic with a 1-year history of a black discoloration and nail changes to the tip of his left thumb.

Description of the Problem

The patient has a high probability of having a subungual malignant melanoma. There is a high level of surgical urgency because of the aggressiveness of the tumor.

Key Anatomy

Melanoma is a malignant cancer of the skin that develops from melanocytes. It is particularly aggressive. The prognosis is based on the depth of the tumor. Two classification schemes are frequently used. One is the Breslow classification, which measures, in millimeters, the thickness of the depth of invasion. A thickness of 0.75-millimeter or less usually carries an excellent prognosis. The prognosis worsens as the thickness increases. Patients with lesions thicker than 4 mm have a survival rate of less than 50%. The second classification is the Clark classification. It has five levels and is an anatomic classification based on the involvement of various depths of the epidermis, the dermis, and the subcutaneous tissue. For example, level 1 involves only the epidermis, with no invasion into the dermis. Levels 2 through 4 show progressive invasion of the papillary and the reticular dermis. Level 5 melanomas invade the subcutaneous tissue.

Workup

A patient presenting with discoloration of the nail requires prompt attention. A detailed history is helpful. For example, recent trauma to the nail by a crush injury may have caused a localized subungual hematoma that will clear over time. However, if the history is unclear or if the lesion arose some time ago, then the most prudent plan is to perform an incisional biopsy. Missing a melanoma diagnosis is catastrophic.

Treatment

The nail is removed, and a full-thickness incisional biopsy is performed, with markings of the orientation of the tissue. The nail can be replaced as a splint of the nail fold. If the pathology returns as a melanoma, then the local tumor board should fully evaluate the patient for all treatment options. In this case of a malignant melanoma involving the subungual tissue, the safest treatment is amputation. If a tumor is localized in the subungual tissue, then usually an interphalangeal joint disarticulation is sufficient. However, in this case, the discoloration of the tumor spreads proximal to the interphalangeal joint; therefore a more proximal amputation at the mid to distal proximal phalanx is necessary to clear the skin of color changes.

The specimen is carefully reviewed in pathology for removal of the tumor. In most cases of extremity melanoma, a sentinel node biopsy is required. This will identify any nodes in the elbow or axilla that may be involved in the tumor. Systemic treatment is needed if any of these nodes are positive. The patient is followed by a medical oncologist for possible treatment with interferon or another chemotherapeutic modality.

Alternatives

There are no treatment alternatives to this very aggressive cancer. Some authors will attempt to save the distal phalanx, because only the skin is involved. This is a risk that most surgeons and patients do not wish to take.

Principles and Clinical Pearls

- Any discoloration under the nails must alert hand surgeons to the possibility of malignant melanoma.
- Understanding the various classifications of melanoma depth is essential.
- Aggressive treatment with amputation and sentinel node biopsy with follow-up in the medical oncology clinic is critical to save this patient.

Pitfalls

The main pitfall is related to misdiagnosing the tumor. Medical personnel must be hypervigilant to the possibility of melanoma at all times. Subungual melanomas are very lethal, because they are often missed.

Classic References

Ito T, Wada M, Nagae K, Nakano-Nakamura M, Nakahara T, Hagihara A, Furue M, Uchi H. Acral lentiginous melanoma: who benefits from sentinel lymph node biopsy? J Am Acad Dermatol 72:71, 2015.
This was a recent retrospective review of 116 patients who underwent sentinel lymph node biopsy for acral lentiginous melanoma. The authors are beginning to define the indications for sentinel node biopsy.

Nguyen J, Bakri K, Nguyen EC, Johnson CH, Moran SL. Surgical management of subungual melanoma: Mayo clinic experience of 124 cases. Ann Plast Surg 71:346, 2013.
This was a large series of 124 cases of surgical management of subungual melanoma. It was an excellent review of treatment, including amputation, disease progression, and survival analysis.

98 Schwannoma

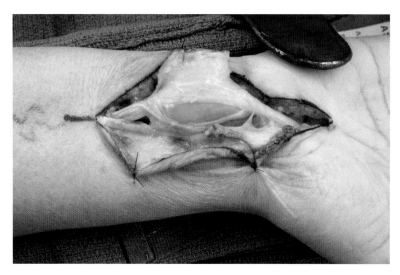

This woman is seen intraoperatively with a median nerve mass.

Description of the Problem

The patient has had tingling in the median nerve distribution and a mass in the distal volar forearm for the past several years. Light touch led to electrical shocks in the median nerve distribution. An MRI showed a mass within the median nerve. The patient has a nerve mass of unknown cause.

Key Anatomy

The median nerve in the distal forearm proceeds distally into the carpal canal and then branches into motor functions controlling the intrinsic muscles of the thumb and sensation to the thumb, the index finger, the middle finger, and half of the ring finger. It is critical for hand function.

Workup

The initial presentation showed a mass in the distal forearm with median nerve symptoms. In this area, the mass could be any type of hand and upper extremity tumor. Because there are median nerve symptoms, it is important to assess the function of the median nerve in terms of volar abduction of the thumb and thumb intrinsic muscle strength and bulk. Sensation is carefully documented.

Palpating the mass can help to determine whether it is freely movable. Tapping on the mass will reveal nerve symptoms such as a Tinel sign. An MRI is needed to assess nerve involvement because of the critical nature of the nerve function. Classically an MRI will show a well-circumscribed mass in the nerve itself. Consent should be carefully obtained for treatment needed for a schwannoma or a neurofibroma. Patients with extensive nerve involvement should provide consent for nerve resection and immediate nerve grafting.

An intraoperative dissection revealed intact fascicles and a normal nerve proximal and distal to the mass; the fascicles could be dissected to one involved fascicle with the mass. The mass is probably a schwannoma, because it was easily dissected free from the remainder of the mass.

Treatment

A schwannoma can be carefully dissected down to one fascicle that can be removed with minimal impact on the overall nerve function. This is the most critical part of treatment. Often, hand surgeons are presented with a patient who has already undergone a biopsy procedure for a schwannoma. This is a devastating occurrence, because a random biopsy may obliterate the normal tissue planes within the nerve and lead to severe nerve deficits. In the operation, normal nerve needs to be identified proximally and distally and the operating microscope used to carefully tease out the fascicles until the mass can be isolated on one fascicle, which is removed.

Alternatives

The only alternative to careful microsurgical resection is to leave the mass alone. However, patients usually have nerve symptoms such as an irritating sensitivity and tingling. As the mass grows, it can compress the rest of the nerve and cause nerve deficits.

Principles and Clinical Pearls

- In cases of suspected nerve tumors, careful preoperative imaging is critical.
- A schwannoma can be meticulously dissected free from the rest of nerve, and most nerve function can be preserved.
- Other nerve tumors may not be easily dissected free; therefore nerve reconstruction with nerve grafting may be necessary.

Pitfalls

All pitfalls relate to misdiagnosis. Haphazard dissection, unnecessary nerve resection, and poor technique will lead to nerve deficits.

Classic Reference

Gosk J, Gutkowska O, Mazurek P, Koszewicz M, Ziółkowski P. Peripheral nerve tumours: 30-year experience in the surgical treatment. Neurosurg Rev 38:511, 2015.

This review article presented a 30-year experience with surgical treatment of peripheral nerve tumors. Most of the tumors were benign, and nerve function was preserved with careful dissection.

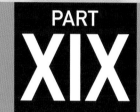

PART

XIX

Vascular Conditions

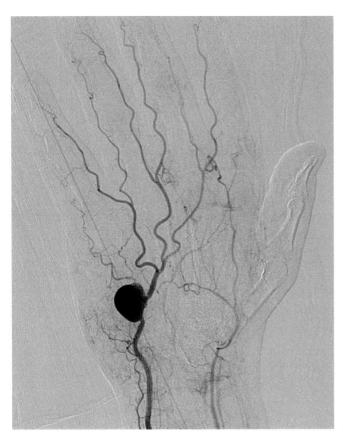

This is an angiogram of a patient with a palpable, pulsatile mass in his right palm. This is beginning to affect his work as a mechanic. The patient notes episodic numbness and purplish discoloration at the tips of his ring and small fingers. The fingertips are noticeably cooler than those on the other side.

Description of the Problem

The patient has a hypothenar hammer syndrome, with a large aneurysm involving the ulnar artery as it exits the Guyon canal. The aneurysm has decreased flow with sludging of the blood and evidence of partial thrombosis of the aneurysm cavity. The palmar arch is incomplete, with minimal flow from the radial artery. The patient is at risk for thrombosis of the ulnar artery, clot formation, and distal emboli. He has ulnar nerve symptoms consisting of intrinsic weakness and numbness of the ring and small fingers.

Key Anatomy

The radial and ulnar arteries contribute to the perfusion to the hand. The radial artery forms a deep carpal arch with primary blood flow to the radial side of the hand. The ulnar artery exits the Guyon canal and forms the superficial arch. Most patients have two interconnected vascular networks involving the deep palmar arch from the radial artery and the superficial palmar arch from the ulnar artery. In this patient's angiogram, flow to the deep arch is minimal, and no connections exist between the ulnar and radial sides of the hand. Therefore, if this ulnar artery aneurysm and thrombosis clots off, the patient will have severely limited blood flow to the fingers.

Workup

Patients usually present with episodic discoloration and numbness to the tips of the fingers. A pulsatile, painful mass may be noted in the palm of the hand. Intrinsic weakness and numbness to the ring and small fingers may be present because the mass compresses the ulnar nerve in the Guyon canal. After a careful physical examination and an Allen test are completed, vascular imaging is usually required. An angiogram is the benchmark modality. For patients who cannot tolerate an angiogram because of dye allergies, an MR angiogram may be a substitute diagnostic test. Although other tests such as digital plethysmography and Doppler and duplex ultrasound may be proposed, an angiogram is the best test, because it shows the entire road map of the hand.

Treatment

Treatment depends on the availability of collateral blood flow. This patient has minimal flow from the radial artery; therefore the ulnar artery aneurysm should be excised and the ulnar artery reconstructed. This is performed using microsurgical technique. The Guyon tunnel is released with a longitudinal incision, and the ulnar nerve is protected. The ulnar artery aneurysm is carefully dissected, and good proximal and distal control of the ulnar artery is achieved. This is performed under an operating microscope. The aneurysm is excised, and the ends of the ulnar artery are carefully evaluated. If sufficient laxity is noted in the usually tortuous ulnar artery, it may be possible to perform an end-to-end anastomosis of the ulnar artery. However, a short vein graft may be needed, harvested from either the hand or foot. The graft should not be too long, because it could kink at the ulnar artery level. Once blood flow is restored, the hand is evaluated, and the wound is closed.

Alternatives

Some authors have advocated simply ligating the ulnar artery to prevent distal emboli. This patient lacks collateral flow from the radial side, and ulnar artery reconstruction is critical.

Principles and Clinical Pearls

- An angiogram is the benchmark for evaluating vascular abnormalities involving the hand.
- Microsurgical technique is critical for this case. Surgeons should understand the relative contributions of the radial and ulnar arteries to the blood flow to the hand. If the arch is incomplete, every effort must be made to reconstruct the ulnar artery.
- The ulnar nerve, especially the deep motor branch, should be protected.

Pitfalls

Pitfalls are common to any microsurgical technique. They include thrombosis of the microsurgical anastomosis and other technical problems. The ulnar nerve needs to be protected.

Classic References

Hui-Chou HG, McClinton MA. Current options for treatment of hypothenar hammer syndrome. Hand Clin 31:53, 2015.
Dr. McClinton's group is well known for microvascular reconstruction of the hand. This review article was an excellent evaluation of the methods for optimal treatment of hypothenar hammer syndrome.

Yuen JC, Wright E, Johnson LA, Culp WC. Hypothenar hammer syndrome: an update with algorithms for diagnosis and treatment. Ann Plast Surg 67:429, 2001.
This excellent review of hypothenar hammer syndrome included photographs showing the anatomy and pathophysiology of this condition. Algorithms were proposed for optimal treatment.

100 Scleroderma

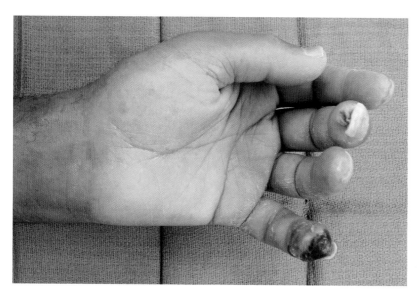

This patient is seen in the clinic with necrosis at the tips of her middle and small fingers. She has a history of scleroderma. She notes cold intolerance, pain in her hands, and nonhealing wounds.

Description of the Problem

The patient has manifestations of scleroderma. This is an autoimmune disease of the connective tissue. The cause is unknown. It is characterized by fibrosis of the skin and internal organs with involvement of multiple organs, including the gastrointestinal tract, the heart, the lungs, the kidneys, and the musculoskeletal system. Scleroderma is also known as *systemic sclerosis*. CREST syndrome includes *c*alcinosis, *R*aynaud phenomenon, *e*sophageal dysmotility, *s*cleroderma, and *t*elangiectasia. Systemic sclerosis of the hand has three main components: digital ischemia with skin changes, calcinosis, and joint contractures. All of these hand manifestations may require a hand surgery evaluation and treatment.

Key Anatomy

The relevant anatomy is related to the three manifestations of scleroderma. With digital ischemia, the radial and ulnar arteries have circumferential fibrosis, leading to narrowed vessels. Narrowing of the lumen and thrombosis develop. The deep and superficial arches, the common digital arteries, and the proper digital arteries may be involved in similar progressive narrowing and thrombosis. This leads to Raynaud phenomenon, hand pain, and digital ulcers. The second manifestation of scleroderma, calcinosis, involves excessive calcium deposits in the fingertips. Calcium is deposited throughout the fibrous tissue of the fingertip pulp and causes exquisite pain. The third manifestation of scleroderma is joint contractures. These patients will develop extension contractures of the metacarpophalangeal joints and flexion contractures of the proximal interphalangeal joints.

Workup

A workup for these patients involves a comprehensive review by dermatologists, rheumatologists, and hand surgeons. The systemic manifestations of scleroderma must be controlled with various rheumatologic medications. For a hand surgery workup, radiographs are obtained to assess for evidence of joint contractures. A workup for digital ischemia includes noninvasive techniques, but an angiogram will be required to provide a road map for the hand. The radiographs can reveal areas of calcinosis, because calcium deposits are radiopaque.

Treatment

Medical management, including calcium channel blockers and other medications, should be optimized before all surgical treatments. Digital ischemia is the first problem addressed. The angiogram is reviewed in anticipation of surgery. A sympathectomy may be performed through longitudinal incisions over the radial and ulnar arteries at the level of the wrist, a transverse incision in the palm, and a longitudinal incision in the dorsal snuffbox. The radial and ulnar arteries can be accessed through these incisions. A microscopic sympathectomy includes removal of all sympathetic branches entering these arteries and removal of the fibrosis surrounding the vessels. This is performed through a palm incision. The superficial arch and common digit arteries are accessed. The overall goal of a sympathectomy is to remove the sympathetic inflow, to strip the vessels of periarterial fibrosis, and to assess for the possibility of bypass grafting. Blood flow is greatly increased with a vascular bypass, provided one is possible. The fingertip ulcers can be treated by surgical debridement. Some patients have calcinosis, which can be removed through longitudinal incisions in the pulps of the fingers. There is a fine balance between incisions and healing of the wound. Therefore calcinosis incisions should be minimal. Finally, joint contractures in scleroderma are very difficult to treat. Soft tissue procedures such as a capsulotomy probably will not improve the range of motion. A proximal interphalangeal joint fusion is the preferred treatment for severe flexion deformity of this joint.

Alternatives

The injection of botulinum toxin is an alternative to a sympathectomy. Recent reports show some efficacy for increasing blood flow in these complex patients.

Principles and Clinical Pearls

- Scleroderma patients are extremely complex, and medical management must be optimized before surgical treatment.
- Sympathectomy has been shown to be very beneficial for increasing blood flow. However, these patients will never have normal blood flow, and blood flow may worsen over time.
- Calcinosis excision can decrease pain; joint fusion can improve the posture of the hand.

Pitfalls

Scleroderma patients are extremely complex and carry a high surgical risk. Pulmonary function and kidney function must be carefully assessed before general anesthesia is given. Wound healing is a concern in patients with distal ischemia; therefore incisions are made judiciously. Last, although sympathectomy has shown good results, blood flow will never be normal.

Classic References

Fox P, Chung L, Chang J. Management of the hand in systemic sclerosis. J Hand Surg Am 38:1012, 2013.
This was a recent review of the management of the hand in systemic sclerosis with specific treatments of digital ischemia, calcinosis, and joint contractures.

Hartzell TL, Makhni EC, Sampson C. Long-term results of periarterial sympathectomy. J Hand Surg Am 34:1454, 2009.
The authors reviewed their experience with periarterial sympathectomy, comparing patients with scleroderma versus patients with other mixed connective tissue disorders. They showed that a periarterial sympathectomy was much more effective in patients with scleroderma, because periarterial fibrosis was addressed.

Index

Radius fracture, 39, 99-100, 103-104, 105-106, 107-108,
   109-110
Raynaud phenomenon, 249
Reduction; *see* Closed reduction; Open reduction
Replantation, thumb, 3-4
Reverse Colles fracture, 107-108
Reverse pedicle radial forearm flap, 240
Reverse radial forearm fasciocutaneous flap, 152
Rheumatoid arthritis
   interphalangeal joint osteoarthritis and, 32
   metacarpophalangeal joint, 35-36
   metacarpophalangeal joint osteoarthritis and, 29
"Rosebud" hands, 69

S

Saddle syndrome, 202
Sagittal band rupture, 161-162
Sauve-Kapandji procedure, 42
Scaphoid excision, 34, 126
Scaphoid fracture, 123-124
Scaphoid nonunion, 125-126
Scapholunate advanced collapse wrist arthritis, 33-34
Scapholunate ligament tear, 159-160
Scaphotrapeziotrapezoid joint osteoarthritis, 27-28
Scar release, in burns, 47-48
Schwannoma, 201, 243-244
Scleroderma, 249-250
Secondary intention, healing by, 13, 138
Septic arthritis
   in cat bite injury, 136
   in human bite injury, 134
   in paronychia, 137, 138
Shingles, 172
Shoulder arthrodesis, in brachial plexus injury, 190
Skin cancer, 239-240, 241-242
Skin graft
   in exposed flexor tendon, 197
   in syndactyly release, 61-62
   in thermal burn, 45-46
Smith fracture, 107-108
Snow-Littler procedure, 68
"Spade" hands, 69
Spaghetti wrist, 213-214
Spastic hand and wrist contractures, 77-78
Spiral oblique retinacular ligament reconstruction, 216
Splinting
   in boutonnière deformity, 217, 218
   in carpal tunnel syndrome, 170
   in cubital tunnel syndrome, 173
   in de Quervain tenosynovitis, 204
   in fingertip defect repair, 12
   in hand burn, 45-46
   in interphalangeal joint osteoarthritis, 29

   in mallet finger, 219-220
   in metacarpophalangeal joint osteoarthritis, 29
   in pisotriquetral joint osteoarthritis, 37
   in posttraumatic wrist arthritis, 40
   in proximal interphalangeal joint dislocation frac-
      ture, 117-118
   in radial tunnel syndrome, 177
   in scaphoid nonunion, 126
   in scapholunate advanced collapsed wrist arthritis,
      34
   in scaphotrapeziotrapezoid joint osteoarthritis, 28
   in swan-neck deformity, 216
   in thumb carpometacarpal joint osteoarthritis, 25
   in thumb replantation, 4
   in trigger finger, 201
   in ulnar nerve palsy, 185
   in Wartenberg syndrome, 21
"Spoon" hands, 69
Squamous cell carcinoma, 239-240
Staged flexor tendon reconstruction, 225-227
Static capsulodesis, in scapholunate ligament tear, 160
Stener lesions, 158
Stiff finger
   in extension, 79-80
   in flexion, 81-82
Stretching; *see* Passive stretching
Stroke, contracture in, 77
Styloscaphoid arthritis, 33-34
Superficialis to profundus transfer, 78
Superficial palmar arch, in hand near-amputation, 6
Supraclavicular plexus, in brachial plexus injury, 190
Suprascapular nerve, in brachial plexus injury, 190
Swan-neck deformity, 215-216
Sympathectomy, 250
Syndactyly, 61
Syndactyly release, 61-62
   in Apert syndrome, 70
Systemic sclerosis, 249-250

T

Telangiectasia, 249
Tendoligamentous reconstruction, in scapholunate
      ligament tear, 160
Tendon graft
   in flexor tendon adhesions, 223-224
   in sagittal band rupture, 161
   in staged flexor tendon reconstruction, 226
   in swan-neck deformity, 216
Tendon transfer
   in high median and ulnar nerve palsy, 188
   in median nerve palsy, 183
   in radial nerve palsy, 180-181
   in ulnar nerve palsy, 185, 186